Fit Focused Ready

The Guide to Life-Changing Fitness

Bo Bland

Title: Fit Focused Ready: The Guide to Life-Changing Fitness

Author: Bo Bland

Edition: First Edition, 2023

Website: www.FitFocusedReady.com

QR Code for www.fitfocusedready.com

The information provided in this book is for educational and informational purposes only. The views and opinions expressed in this book are those of the author and do not necessarily reflect the official policy or position of any other agency, organization, employer, or company. The author and publisher are not responsible for any specific health or allergy needs that may require medical supervision and are not liable for any damages or negative consequences from any treatment, action, application, or preparation, to any person reading or following the information in this book.

Printed in the United States of America

"Knowing is not enough, we must apply. Willing is not enough, we must do."

Bruce Lee

Contents

- Step 3: No Eating Out: Strategies for avoiding dining out and focusing on home-cooked meals.
- Step 4: Getting Active: Aligning diet with physical activity.
- Step 5: Weekends Are Free: Balancing discipline with flexibility.
- Step 6: Be Mindful: Integrating mindfulness into eating habits.
- Conclusion: Summing up the diet approach and its benefits.

Chapter 1: The Foundation of Transformation

Welcome to Fit Focused Ready: The Guide to Life-Changing Fitness. I'm Bo Bland, the author and creator of this system. I've spent over 15 years analyzing my own thoughts, learning, and refining this system through a lot of trial and error, testing what worked and what didn't. The original intention of this system was to make me a stronger athlete while creating a simple but effective way of eating and exercising to help me in my pursuit of becoming an Ironman Triathlete and a 100-mile ultrarunner. And it worked! So well, in fact, that I wanted to share it with the rest of the world in the hopes that others could see as amazing results as I did.

Nothing here will shatter the world, I promise you. But my approach to fitness is, I guess you could say, wider. What I mean by that is, if you take a step back and look at fitness as a whole, three things stand out. The first two are the simple things: diet and exercise. The last one, which makes the biggest difference, is the mind. But don't get scared; I'm not going all Dalai Lama and Tony Robbins on you. I'm not throwing shade at the Dalai Lama or Tony, but my approach is different. The mind game, to me, is very straightforward and functional. It's more about gaining awareness and control than anything else. But more on that later.

When you take all three pieces—the Diet, the Fitness, and the Mental—and put them together, you get a complete picture, and you finally get to see fitness the way it should be.

How Everything Started: My Story - The Bar Bet That Flipped My World Upside Down

In 2009, there I was: Bo Bland, 25 years old, horribly out of shape (double chin and all), despite seemingly leading an active lifestyle. I was chain-smoking far too many cigarettes, living off junk food, and binge drinking as if it were a competitive sport. Unbeknownst to me, my life and health were spiraling downward.

Then, one night at the bar, amidst slamming back shots and round after round, a friend laid down a challenge in the form of a triathlon. Being who I am, I couldn't resist a good bet – especially one that seemed ridiculously unachievable. Three drunks racing in a triathlon? Count me in. Accepting that triathlon challenge marked a pivotal moment. Little did I know, it would nudge my life onto an entirely new trajectory.

Fast forward to the next day: I was sitting at the computer in my parents' house, staring at what I was about to sign up for: The Assateague Assault Sprint Triathlon. I had just discovered that a triathlon was quite the event: first you swim, then you bike, then you run, all without stopping. That didn't seem right to me, so I called my friend Billy to make sure there wasn't some confusion. Three guys who smoke and get drunk every weekend, and had been doing so for over 8 years, should not even be considering a race like this. But he assured me that yes, that's what we were doing. So, I did what any other reckless person might do—I said, "F#ck it," and signed up.

Over the next few weeks and months, my training was minimal at best. I ran sporadically, but found it so unenjoyable that I adhered to a 'less is more' strategy. Similarly, my efforts on the bike were half-hearted, as I found biking challenging and not particularly enjoyable.

Before delving further, let me tell you about my bike. I chose a red, early '90s Diamondback Ascent EX mountain bike for this adventure. It was my father's, having been stored under their house for the last decade. It seemed perfect for the job, but in reality, it was far from it. The bike was slightly too big, the seat was incredibly uncomfortable, and the tires were dry-rotted. The gears didn't shift well either. My makeshift solution? I balled up a sweatshirt, taped it to the seat to spare my discomfort, and pumped up the tires. I decided to simply ignore the rest of the problems. So, with the bike 'sorted,' it was time to address swimming.

Having lived near water most of my life, I had always been comfortable swimming. However, training for distance swimming was a new and daunting challenge. During my first attempt at swim training, I realized my grave mistake. I had never actually tried to swim any significant distance. Barely 50 feet into my swim, I was exhausted and gasping for air at the edge of the local swim center's pool. Puzzled, I wondered, "How long is this swim, and how many laps do I need to complete?" After some research, I learned that the swim portion of the Assateague Assault Sprint Triathlon was a half-mile, equating to about 16 laps of an Olympic pool. This was discouraging news, considering I was struggling to complete even half a lap.

Moreover, I couldn't swim freestyle with my face in the water. Each time I tried, I ended up swallowing a ton of water and choking. It was clear that my swimming technique, slow and exhausting as it was, would have to suffice. I had no other option. My only hope lay in my wetsuit. While I might not have been able to swim efficiently, I certainly could float. The buoyancy of the wetsuit ensured that I wouldn't sink. With the fear of drowning out of the equation, I felt I could at least float my way to the end of the swim segment.

Then came race day, and it was time to put all my training, or lack thereof, to the test. I arrived on race morning just as the sun began to rise. Parking my truck with the mountain bike in the back, I started looking for my friends. It didn't take long to find them; they were the only ones standing around smoking cigarettes. "Have a smoke?" Of course! We joked about not having a chance of winning and laughed about how awful the race was going to be, already planning our drinks for later.

Seeing their bikes, I had a moment of realization: their bikes were legitimate road bikes. In contrast, my red mountain bike was in poor shape and stood no chance against theirs. Despite this, we joked a bit more and then got down to business, getting ready for the race. As I watched my friends pump up their bike tires, it never occurred to me that I should do the same. In fact, I hadn't added any air to the tires since dragging the bike out from under my parents' house. This oversight in critical thinking would come back to haunt me later in the race.

It was time to set up our transition area. In a triathlon, the transition area is where you rack your bike and place items like your bike helmet, running shoes, a towel, and anything else you might need during the race, such as food or drink. It's where you switch from one portion of the race to the next. With my transition area ready, I put on my wetsuit and started walking down to the beach to begin the race.

As my friends and I walked and talked, the reality of the distance began to dawn on me. We had been walking a long time, and the swim seemed daunting. Despite growing doubt, I tried to keep my cool. As the race director announced "60 seconds to race start" through a bullhorn, my heart pounded. I wished for everything to just stop, but no such luck. The airhorn sounded, and we all dashed into the ocean.

Chaos ensued, with waves crashing and swimmers colliding. There was kicking, punching, and goggles being pulled off in a frenzied melee. I struggled to keep calm and swim through it all. About eight minutes later, I reached open water and the first buoy. It was time to start the half-mile swim. Initially relieved to be clear of the chaos, I soon found myself in trouble. Exhausted, I resorted to treading water. My secret weapon? The backstroke, which was essentially just me floating on my back, kicking my legs, and making an awkward frog-like motion with my arms. This was my plan to complete the swim.

However, about five to ten minutes into my backstroke, a lifeguard on a paddleboard paddled over and informed me, "Hey man! You are swimming in circles!" Barely able to see through fogged-up goggles, I muttered a weak "okay, thanks." My strategy had failed, and I had no choice but to swim as best I could towards the beach. I alternated between swimming, floating, and resting, feeling both exhausted and miserable, but I was making progress. Finally, after 30 minutes, the swim was over. Stumbling up the beach, I was relieved it was done. Seeing my mother cheering me on lifted my spirits as I made my way to the transition area.

Removing a wetsuit in a triathlon is a challenge in itself. My arms were already dead tired, and the suit clung stubbornly to my body. With assistance from a spectator, I eventually managed to peel it off. After a quick sip of water, I donned my sunglasses, bike shoes, and helmet, grabbed my bike, and started the bike portion of the race.

Initially, things seemed to be going well; I was moving along, grateful to no longer be swimming. However, it wasn't long before the situation deteriorated. I was not only exhausted but also incredibly thirsty, and I had no water. I hadn't realized that bringing water was an option, and my bike lacked a water cage holder anyway. Pushing through, I realized about five miles into the 13-mile bike course that my tires were nearly flat. Each pedal push made the tires squash down, making it feel like I was biking through quicksand, draining my already depleted energy. Then, unexpectedly, one of my friends – apparently an even worse swimmer than I was – caught up and swiftly passed me with a quick "Hey, Bo," disappearing into the distance. I had no chance of catching up, but I kept pushing forward and eventually reached the end of the bike portion. Relieved, I racked my bike, switched to my running shoes, chugged some water, and began the running segment.

Running in a triathlon is akin to running on legs that feel like a mix of Jello and cement. They wobble and resist every move. For the first half-mile, catching my breath was a struggle, necessitating frequent stops and walks, almost every 20 feet. Then, something remarkable happened. Somehow, inexplicably, I found my rhythm and could run. I managed to maintain a decent pace without feeling on the brink of collapse. It was challenging, yes, but manageable. Suddenly, I had completed mile one, then two, and before I knew it, mile three. Only 0.1 mile remained to the finish line. Rounding a turn, I sprinted down the straightaway and crossed the finish line. It was over. I was exhausted, but I had done it. We spent the rest of the afternoon recounting the race's challenges and laughing over its absurdities, yet we all agreed it was fun.

Fast forward a few months, and my lifestyle hadn't changed much. The drinking and poor diet persisted, but something within me had shifted. I wasn't the same person anymore. There was talk of participating in another race, but nothing concrete materialized. Time passed.

The genesis of the next chapter in my journey is a bit hazy, but it involved a conversation with my dad about the Marine Corps Marathon, a race he had completed the previous year. I'm not sure how the conversation went, but I found myself agreeing to run the Marine Corps Marathon and to attempt the Assateague Assault Sprint Triathlon once more. There was no denying it – something about the challenge was invigorating, and I was drawn to the sense of accomplishment it brought.

By early summer 2010, my father and I had recently completed the Assateague Assault Sprint Triathlon, and my performance had improved significantly. We were gearing up to start training for the marathon in the fall. It was then that I realized running was my forte. While I struggled with biking and swimming, running was a different story – I was actually quite good at it and found myself increasingly enjoying it. A few runs into our training program, my father handed me a book: "Ultra Marathon Man" by Dean Karnazes. The book was a revelation. Here was a man running through the night, traversing mountains and deserts, completing 100 and 200-mile races, and he was an Ironman too. The concept of running such distances was beyond my comprehension. I was captivated and knew right then that I wanted to be an ultra-runner and an Ironman Triathlete. This book changed my outlook on life; I started to think about my diet, strength training, running gear, and triathlon bikes. A goal was set, and I was determined to achieve it.

To say I was undergoing a change would be an understatement. My focus narrowed to nothing but my goal. I trained relentlessly, balancing it with my social life, which meant training on Saturday mornings and partying on Saturday nights. I was young, single, and enjoyed a good time, but regardless of the previous night's activities, I was back to training by Monday morning, or even Sunday if needed. I would run, hungover or sick if necessary. These two lifestyles were at odds, but I managed to make it work through sheer willpower. However, I did make some significant adjustments – I quit smoking and eliminated all junk food from my diet. These changes alone made an immense difference. I felt healthier and more vibrant than ever before.

Though I still hadn't quite figured out the diet aspect. The information out there was confusing, often contradictory. I experimented with an all-meat diet, but quickly realized it wasn't for me, not to mention my aversion to cooking. Then I tried an all-fruit diet, which I absolutely loved. It made my body feel supercharged. However, this diet clashed with my social life. Eating only fruit all week and then drinking all night on Saturdays was a recipe for feeling sick. So, reluctantly, I abandoned the all-fruit diet.

After trying several other diets and finding them lacking, I decided to synthesize what I had learned and create my own dietary system. I named it "Only Good Options." It was simple, effective, and perfectly tailored to my lifestyle, allowing me to enjoy both my social life and my rigorous training for various races.

Early in my training, around the time my dad and I signed up for the marathon, I recognized the importance of strength training. It was crucial not just for aesthetics – though as a single guy, looking good was a bonus – but also for improving my performance in running, biking, and swimming. I wasn't much of a gym enthusiast; I preferred doing strength training at home, focusing on bodyweight exercises. To my surprise, these simple exercises were remarkably effective in keeping me fit and looking good – far from the stereotypical stick figure runner. A few times a week of this routine was all it took. It was simple, yet it worked wonders.

During this period, I was training for marathons, triathlons, and gradually increasing my trail running mileage. Everything culminated in 2013 when I signed up for my first 100-mile ultramarathon – The Leadville 100-mile run, followed a month later by the Panama City Ironman Triathlon. All my training was leading up to these events, and I felt prepared.

Before I even reached these ultra-distance races, I had learned something crucial: the importance of mental strength. From the very beginning, going back to my first triathlon, I realized the immense power of the mind. It can be both manipulative and incredibly strong. I experienced firsthand the difficulty of resisting deep-seated desires or forcing myself out of bed on a cold winter morning for a run in the rain. The mind can be a ruthless adversary, knowing all your weaknesses and exploiting them. Yet, it is also your strongest ally, capable of pushing you to heights you never imagined possible. Delving into my own mind, I learned to harness its power and direct it as I saw fit. It became my greatest strength and most powerful tool.

When I lined up at the start of the Leadville 100 and later at the Panama City Ironman, I knew that while my physical training had brought me this far, it was my mind that would carry me through to the finish. And it did. Crossing those finish lines was the realization of my dreams. Holding those medals, I thought to myself, "That was fun, what's next?" And I haven't stopped since.

In this book, I break down every aspect of my transformation from an out-of-shape drunk to an ultra-runner and Ironman. From mental strength to diet and fitness, I explain how these components work, why they work, and how you can apply them too. The principles I share are foundational; they form the backbone upon which everything else relies. Used correctly, they can simplify your life and elevate you to new heights.

Let's begin:

The Power of the Mind:

Understanding the techniques of mental strength.

It has been said that the mind is a powerful thing; I believe this to be a complete understatement. A dump truck is a powerful thing, but the mind is on a whole different level. Everything you see, everything you do, everything you think, all starts in the mind. Your entire world — how you perceive it and the actions you take — is all dictated by your mind. It has the power to create pure paralyzing fear or a confidence so strong that anything seems possible. I have learned the power of the mind firsthand. It has been my best friend and my worst enemy. I know the lies it can tell and the motivation it can bring.

In this first section of Fit Focused Ready, I will give you all the tools I learned, or more accurately, became aware of, while on my journey to ultrarunner status. Each tool was first used subconsciously, and over time, as I became more aware of my mind's workings, I learned to control it. I mastered how to activate it when needed and to recognize when I was being deceived. This road is not paved with gold; it's hard and will take constant effort. But within the mind, you will find your greatest strength and your greatest weaknesses.

Please note that every tool I will give you I still use to this day. These lifelong tools, if used correctly, will take you further than you ever could have dreamed.

<u>**Tool 1.**</u>

Being Mindful:

Techniques and benefits of mindfulness.

Being mindful isn't just some new age concept, it's a powerful tool that allows us to take control of our thoughts and emotions. It's about being aware of what's going on inside our heads so that we can make better decisions and respond to situations in a more calculated way. By practicing mindfulness, we can take emotions out of the equation and make wiser decisions that align with our goals.

The truth is, emotional wants and negative thoughts can easily derail our progress if we're not careful. That's why it's important to focus on our mental state and keep our thoughts and emotions in check. When we feel an emotional want, fear, or doubt creeping in, we can take a step back, evaluate the situation, and act in a more calculated way.

It takes practice to become more mindful, but the results are worth it. By simply being aware of your emotions as you make decisions throughout your day, you can start to take control of your life and unlock your full potential. It won't happen overnight, but with consistency and dedication, you'll find that being mindful becomes second nature.

One way to become more mindful is to practice mindfulness exercises, which can help you develop the ability to focus your attention on the present moment. This can be as simple as taking a few deep breaths and noticing the sensations in your body or becoming aware of your thoughts without getting lost in them.

The benefits of mindfulness are numerous. Studies have shown that regular mindfulness practice can help reduce stress, improve concentration and focus, and even boost immune function. It can also help you develop greater self-awareness and emotional intelligence, which can lead to more meaningful relationships and a greater sense of well-being.

In terms of achieving your goals, being mindful can be a powerful tool. By staying aware of your thoughts and emotions, you can better understand what's driving your behavior and make more intentional choices. For example, if you're trying to lose weight and you notice that you're feeling stressed or anxious, you might be more likely to reach for unhealthy comfort foods. But if you're aware of your emotions and how they're impacting your choices, you can choose to respond in a different way, such as taking a walk or doing a relaxation exercise instead of turning to food.

So, in summary, being mindful is about being present in the moment and aware of your thoughts and emotions. It can be a powerful tool for achieving your goals and improving your overall well-being.

Real World Example:

Imagine it's another busy Wednesday evening. You're driving home from work, and the familiar hunger pangs set in. This is the moment your mental toolkit from "Fit Focused Ready" springs into action, not just as concepts, but as practical, powerful allies in your quest for health.

First up, mindfulness. As the allure of fast food tempts you, mindfulness steps forward. It's like an old friend, reminding you to pause and recognize what's happening. "Is this hunger or habit?" it asks. You acknowledge the craving, but with mindfulness, you see it for what it is – a temporary urge that doesn't align with your deeper goals.

Then, your mindset shifts gears. This isn't just about denying yourself a quick fix; it's about affirming a commitment to your health. You remember the goals you've set, the progress you've made. This mindset isn't a passive observer; it's an active participant, steering your decisions towards the healthier choice.

<u>**Tool 2.**</u>

Cultivating a Focused Mindset:

Strategies for developing a strong mental approach.

In the realm of physical and mental endurance, your mindset isn't just a part of the game; it is the game. It's where the rubber meets the road, where your goals are either forged into reality or lost in the noise of distraction. So, let's break down what it truly means to harness a focused mindset in the pursuit of fitness and self-transformation.

Your mindset is like a compass, guiding your thoughts, actions, and ultimately, your outcomes. It's what you focus on, consistently and unwaveringly. When it comes to fitness, particularly in realms as demanding as triathlons or ultramarathons, your mindset needs to be as sharp and focused as a laser beam. This isn't about vague aspirations; it's about a crystal-clear picture of what you want to achieve.

To cultivate a powerful fitness mindset, you first need to be mindful. Being mindful is about staying aware and present, recognizing where your thoughts are drifting. It's easy to let your mind wander into the territory of doubt, fear, or exhaustion. Mindfulness is your checkpoint, ensuring you're still on course.

The goal here is to keep your mindset locked onto your fitness objectives. Whether it's completing that extra mile, nailing a new personal best, or simply getting out the door for a workout, your mindset should be rooted in these goals. Every other thought – the fatigue, the discomfort, the temptation to slack off – should be recognized and then gently steered back towards your objective.

Consider your mindset as focused attention. This isn't a passive state; it's active and dynamic. It's about continually reminding yourself of your goals and why they matter. In fitness, this might mean focusing on the feeling of strength you gain with each workout, the sense of achievement in every small win, or the endorphin rush that follows a challenging run.

Your fitness mindset, therefore, is not just about the act of exercising; it's about embracing the entire journey – the training, the discipline, the nutrition, and the recovery. It's about seeing every aspect of this journey as a vital piece of the puzzle, contributing to your overarching goal.

The beauty of mindset is that it's adaptable. While our focus here is fitness, the principles apply universally. A money mindset zeroes in on financial goals; a leadership mindset on influencing and guiding others. By applying the same principles of focused attention and mindfulness, any goal becomes more attainable.

Real World Example:

Picture this: You're settled in your favorite reading spot with the leadership book in hand. It's a quiet evening, the perfect time to absorb new knowledge. Yet, as you start reading, thoughts about the weekend begin to intrude. Plans, anticipations, the promise of relaxation – all these thoughts start to cloud your focus.

First, you employ mindfulness. It acts like a gentle nudge, bringing your attention back to the present moment. You observe the wandering thoughts without judgment, acknowledging their presence. "Ah, there's me thinking about the weekend again," you note mentally. With this awareness, you gently steer your attention back to the book. Mindfulness isn't about forcefully pushing thoughts away; it's about recognizing them and then returning to the task at hand, in this case, reading.

Now, your mindset takes the stage. You remind yourself of the purpose behind this reading session. "I'm here to grow as a leader, to gain skills that will benefit my team and me," you tell yourself. This mindset isn't just a passive state; it's an active choice to prioritize your personal development over fleeting distractions.

Every time your thoughts stray to the weekend, you use mindfulness to acknowledge and let go of these distractions. Then, your mindset reaffirms your commitment to learning and growth. It's like a cycle: mindfulness brings you back, and your mindset reinforces your purpose.

As you get deeper into the book, you find that the practice of returning your focus becomes more natural. Your mind starts to engage with the content, drawing connections to your own experiences and future aspirations as a leader.

<u>**Tool 3.**</u>

Self-Visualization of the Present:

Techniques for visualizing.

Visualize The New You - The Present

How do you see yourself when you close your eyes? A strong, fit, confident success, or someone battling insecurities and dissatisfaction? Your self-visualization — this mental image you have — profoundly impacts your life, your actions, even your speech. It shapes your beliefs, attitudes, and behaviors, influencing your life's outcomes. If you view yourself as a victor, you're more likely to act toward success. Conversely, seeing yourself as a loser might lead you to settle for less.

The great news? You can change this visualization. By picturing yourself with all the qualities and successes you desire, you transform your beliefs and behaviors, turning dreams into reality. This book will guide you to create a vivid, emotionally-charged image of your desired self. You'll learn to conquer limiting beliefs and doubts, and apply this powerful self-visualization towards achieving your goals, be it in your career, relationships, health, or happiness.

So, take a deep breath, close your eyes, and let's start visualizing the new you.

The Power of Perception

Your perception profoundly influences your approach to life. How you see yourself impacts your decisions, actions, and outcomes. Perception is not objective reality; it's shaped by experiences, culture, conditioning, and beliefs. It's subjective and personal.

Your self-perception affects every life aspect, including relationships, career, and health. Positive self-view breeds optimism and confidence, paving the way for success. Negative perception, however, can lead to discouragement and failure. But you have the power to change this. Through self-visualization, you can positively alter your self-perception. By consistently picturing yourself as confident and successful, this image becomes your reality.

Visualization is a proven life-transformer. Athletes use it to enhance performance, and it applies to all life areas. Understanding and practicing self-visualization can change your beliefs and behaviors, leading you to achieve your goals.

Creating Your Ideal Self: A Step-by-Step Guide

Step 1: Define Your Ideal Self

Know what you want. What does your ideal self look like? What kind of person do you aspire to be? Detail these qualities.

Step 2: Visualize

Close your eyes. Picture this ideal version of yourself in various scenarios — at work, with friends, exercising. Make it vivid.

Step 3: Engage Your Senses

In your visualization, incorporate all senses. For example, as an ultra-trail runner, I picture my dream trail vividly — the mountains, the breeze, the feeling of endurance. This is the power of detailed visualization.

Step 4: Embrace Positivity

Focus on the joy, confidence, and pride associated with your ideal self. Let these feelings fuel your visualization.

Step 5: Repeat

Make this a daily practice. Embed this visualization in your subconscious, aligning your actions with your ideal self.

Overcoming Limiting Beliefs

We all have limiting beliefs that can hold us back. The first step is awareness. When negative thoughts arise, question them. Are they facts or beliefs? Challenge these beliefs and replace them with empowering ones, like "I am capable of achieving my goals." This shift from limiting to empowering beliefs transforms your self-visualization and life.

Real World Example:

Imagine it's early morning and you're standing in front of the mirror, gearing up for a challenging day at work followed by a workout session. This is the perfect moment for the tool of Self-Visualization of the Present to come into play. You take a deep breath and look at your reflection, not just at the surface level, but deeper, into the person you aspire to be.

In this moment of reflection, you start visualizing yourself as the embodiment of the qualities you strive for. You see a confident, resilient professional, ready to tackle any work challenge with poise and determination. You visualize handling difficult tasks, engaging in productive meetings, and contributing innovatively to your projects. This isn't just wishful thinking; it's an affirmation of your capabilities and potential.

You then shift the visualization towards the latter part of your day. You see yourself at the gym, not just going through the motions, but fully engaged in your workout. You visualize yourself pushing through the last difficult reps, maintaining perfect form, and feeling the satisfaction of a workout well done. This visualization is a powerful reinforcement that you are not just dreaming of physical fitness and professional success – you are actively stepping into those roles.

As you step out for the day, these visualizations act like a mental armor. They remind you that you are capable, strong, and ready to rise to the challenges of the day. Each positive action and decision you make throughout the day further cements this self-visualization, turning it from a morning exercise into a living reality. You are not just imagining the person you want to be; you are actively becoming that person, step by step, choice by choice.

Tool 4.

Self-Visualization of the Future:

The power of the future you.

Self-visualization of the Future – The Future You

Self-visualization of the future is a powerful technique that can help you achieve your goals and create the life you truly desire. It involves creating a mental picture of the future you, the person you want to become, and visualizing every detail of their life.

When you use self-visualization, you are tapping into the power of your imagination to create a clear and compelling vision of what you want to achieve. You imagine yourself as the person you want to be, with all the qualities, attributes, and successes that come with it. You visualize your future self standing tall, confident, and strong, with the life you've always wanted.

But it's not just about the external details. Self-visualization also involves visualizing the internal aspects of your future self. You visualize how you feel, your level of confidence, your sense of purpose, and your happiness. You see yourself as someone who has achieved their goals and is living a life of fulfillment and joy.

When you use self-visualization of the future, you are creating a powerful belief in yourself and your abilities. You are putting emotion behind that belief, which helps to solidify it in your mind. The more you can see yourself as that future person, the more likely you are to believe that it's possible and take the necessary steps to make it a reality.

This visualization technique is like a daydream, but with intention. You are intentionally creating a mental picture of your future self and using it as a guide for your daily actions. You have so much confidence in your future self that it guides your steps, giving you the motivation and drive to take the necessary action to achieve your goals.

So, if you want to create the life you truly desire, start visualizing your future self today. Imagine yourself as the person you want to be, and visualize every detail of your life. Use this mental picture to guide your daily actions and watch as you move closer and closer to the life of your dreams. Remember, with self-visualization, anything is possible!

Real World Example:

Envision this: It's the morning after your triumph, and you're standing on a serene seashore, the gentle waves lapping at your feet, the cool breeze whispering around you.

As you close your eyes, you immerse yourself in this moment of achievement and reflection. You see yourself there, standing taller, imbued with the confidence and satisfaction of someone who has just conquered a major milestone. The air feels different here, filled with a sense of accomplishment and the sweet relief of success. You can almost taste the salt in the air, a symbol of the tears of effort and joy that brought you to this point.

In your mind's eye, you replay the journey that led you here. The early mornings, the late nights, the moments of doubt, and the bursts of breakthrough – all these flash before you like scenes from a movie. But unlike a movie, this is your story, a narrative crafted by your dedication and perseverance.

You feel the weight of the effort it took to reach this goal, but more than that, you feel the lightness of fulfillment. This moment is more than just an end; it's a gateway to new beginnings. As you gaze out at the horizon, where the sea meets the sky, you start to contemplate, "What's next?"

This future self-visualization is a powerful motivator. It's not just a daydream; it's a blueprint for your aspirations. It's a reminder that every step you take in the present is a step towards this moment on the seashore. Each challenge faced, each obstacle overcome, is a part of the journey that leads to this point of reflection and triumph.

As you open your eyes and return to the present, you carry with you the image of your future self, standing victorious on the seashore. This image becomes a beacon, guiding your actions and decisions, keeping you anchored to your goals. It's a promise to yourself that the efforts of today are building the success of tomorrow. Each day, as you work towards your goals, remember this visualization of your future self – it's a powerful testament to where your path can lead when you commit to your vision and strive relentlessly towards it.

Tool 5

Self-Visualization – The Ater Ego:

Visualize Your Inner Superhero

At times, we all feel like we are not good enough, whether it's our appearance, strength, fitness, intelligence, courage, or social skills. These thoughts can quickly lead to negativity and fear, causing us to question our ability to move forward, both mentally and physically. If we let our negative self-visualization take over, we can easily give up or shy away, and our hopes and dreams can come crashing down.

But there's a way out of this cycle of negative thinking - Your Inner Superhero! Your alter ego, the perfect version of you. A person who is strong, healthy, and confident, with no fear, pain, or weaknesses. An absolute machine. And that's you. That's your alter ego, who you can tap into whenever you feel beaten down, broken, inadequate or not good enough.

The superhero you, the unstoppable you. Visualize the amazing person in your mind and transform into that person like a bolt of superhero lightning whenever you need it.

We use our alter egos in times of pain, fear, or doubt, when those negative thoughts start to creep in that we can't make it or we're not good enough. That's when we flip on the alter ego switch and turn into the animal that has no fear, no weakness, and won't stop.

The power of the alter ego is almost unimaginable. When it's turned on, everything we dream of doing becomes possible. Even professional athletes, musicians, and other celebrities use alter egos to overcome their own self-doubt and limitations.

Your alter ego is your superhero, the person you meant to be. When you're going through hell, you can flip the switch and become the unstoppable, fearless, and confident person you were always meant to be. You can rise to action and achieve anything you set your mind to.

So close your eyes and visualize your alter ego, your inner superhero. Who is the perfect you? Who is the person you always dreamed of becoming? When you have that image in your mind, you can flip the switch and become that person whenever you need it. Let your superhero power help you overcome any obstacle and become the best version of yourself.

Real World Example:

imagine you're facing the most grueling challenge you've ever encountered. It's a moment teetering on the edge of your limits, where every fiber of your being screams for respite. You feel battered, your resolve waning, a whisper in your mind saying, "I can't go on." This is the crucible, the moment your alter ego is born.

In this crucible, as you teeter on the brink of surrender, something extraordinary happens. You reach deep within and flip an internal switch. Suddenly, you're no longer the person who is overwhelmed and beaten down; you're the embodiment of indomitable will. You transform into your alter ego, a persona that thrives on challenge, that looks adversity in the eye and says with unyielding defiance, "Is that all you've got? Give me more!"

This alter ego is a powerhouse of resilience and strength, forged in the fires of your toughest trials. It's a version of you that is unrecognizable to the shadows of doubt and fatigue. As this persona takes over, you feel a surge of energy, a wellspring of determination that feels almost superhuman. Your muscles no longer ache with fatigue; they burn with the fire of your newfound strength. Your mind, once clouded with thoughts of giving up, is now laser-focused on conquering the task at hand.

You stand taller, breathe deeper, and push forward with a vigor that you didn't know you possessed. Obstacles that seemed insurmountable now appear as mere stepping stones, challenges to be overcome with grit and tenacity. Your alter ego doesn't just carry you through the hardship; it revels in it, turning pain into power, despair into determination.

This self-visualization of your alter ego becomes a transformative tool. It's not a mere fantasy; it's a potent part of your psyche that you can summon in times of need. Whether it's pushing through the final grueling miles of a marathon, enduring the last excruciating minutes of a challenging workout, or overcoming a seemingly impossible hurdle in your personal or professional life, your alter ego is your secret weapon. It's a reminder that within you lies a well of strength that is formidable, a force that can rise to meet any challenge with a fierce battle cry of, "Bring it on!"

Each time you tap into this alter ego, you not only survive the challenge; you grow stronger from it. You learn that your limits are not where you thought they were; they are far beyond. This self-visualization technique becomes a powerful part of your resilience toolkit, a reminder that when the going gets tough, you have within you an unstoppable force ready to rise and conquer.

<u>**Tool 6.**</u>

Belief and Positive Mental Attitude:

Developing a strong belief system and a positive attitude.

Your Mental Attitude

Belief and a positive mental attitude are two of the most important factors in achieving success in life. It may seem like just a catchy phrase, but trust me, it's true. You can accomplish almost anything with these two powerful traits. The combination of belief and positivity can even surpass knowledge and skill. Someone who truly believes they can achieve something and maintains a positive attitude is unstoppable. They can take a defeat, learn from it, and rise up even stronger than before.

Now, let's delve deeper into what these two traits really mean.

Belief typically comes from a combination of past experiences and attitude towards life. When it comes to achieving a goal, belief often starts with an idea, and then grows as you achieve small victories along the way. Every time you achieve a small win, your perspective on what is possible changes, and your belief in yourself grows stronger. It's important to note that these victories don't even have to be directly related to your end goal. What really matters is that they help build your belief in yourself, which is the key to success.

It's important to understand how belief and a positive mental attitude work together to help you achieve your goals. Belief is the foundation upon which your entire pursuit of a goal is built. Without a strong belief in yourself and your ability to achieve your goal, it becomes difficult to take action towards it. Belief is what keeps you going even when things get tough or when you encounter obstacles along the way.

However, belief alone is not enough. It's important to have a positive mental attitude as well. A positive mental attitude allows you to approach challenges and setbacks with optimism and determination. It helps you maintain a sense of hope and possibility even when things seem difficult or impossible. A positive mental attitude also helps you learn from your mistakes and failures, and view them as opportunities for growth and improvement.

Where a positive mental attitude comes from is a bit more complicated, as it's not always clear. Some people seem to be born with it, while others develop it through encouragement from others. However, what we do know is that it's incredibly powerful. A positive attitude can turn a defeat into a lesson learned and propel you forward. It's not always easy to maintain a positive attitude, but it's a skill you can learn. Focus on the bright side of any situation, see every challenge as an opportunity for growth, and celebrate progress no matter how small.

Developing a positive mental attitude is not always easy, but it's a skill that can be learned and improved with practice. One way to cultivate a positive mental attitude is by focusing on gratitude and positivity. Instead of dwelling on negative thoughts and experiences, try to shift your focus towards what you are grateful for and what is going well in your life. You can also surround yourself with positive influences, such as supportive friends or mentors who encourage and motivate you to keep going towards your goals.

In summary, belief and a positive mental attitude work together to help you achieve your goals. Belief provides the foundation for your pursuit of a goal, while a positive mental attitude helps you maintain a sense of hope, optimism, and determination, even in the face of obstacles and setbacks. By cultivating these qualities within yourself, you can overcome challenges and achieve the success you desire.

Real World Example:

Envision yourself facing a situation where success seems distant and challenges loom large. This could be a daunting project at work, a personal goal that feels out of reach, or any scenario where the odds are stacked against you.

At this moment, your inner belief steps into the spotlight. It's a deep, unwavering conviction in your own abilities and potential. This belief isn't blind optimism; it's built on the foundation of your past successes, your skills, and your unique strengths. You remind yourself of the times you've overcome difficulties, the challenges you've already conquered. This history of resilience fuels your belief that you can, indeed, succeed again.

Alongside this robust belief, your Positive Mental Attitude shines brightly. It's like a beacon of hope in a sea of doubt. Instead of focusing on the potential for failure, you shift your perspective to the possibilities of success. You acknowledge the hurdles but view them as opportunities for growth and learning. Your positive attitude isn't about ignoring the difficulties; it's about approaching them with a mindset that seeks solutions and learning experiences.

Now, as you dive into the task at hand, this combination of belief and positivity becomes your driving force. When you encounter a setback, your belief in yourself assures you that this is just a temporary obstacle, not a dead end. Your positive attitude helps you to quickly regroup, find alternate paths, and keep moving forward.

Each small success along the way reinforces your belief. You celebrate these moments, not just for the achievements themselves, but for the evidence they provide of your capabilities. This continuous cycle of belief and positivity creates a self-fulfilling prophecy of sorts. The more you believe in your ability to succeed and maintain a positive outlook, the more likely you are to achieve your goals.

This mindset isn't just beneficial for overcoming challenges; it also enhances your overall well-being. You find yourself more resilient in the face of stress, more creative in problem-solving, and more capable of handling whatever life throws your way.

In essence, the combination of Belief and Positive Mental Attitude is like a dynamic duo within your mental toolkit. It empowers you to face challenges with confidence and optimism, turning potential setbacks into stepping stones towards your success. This approach not only brings you closer to achieving your specific goals but also contributes to a more fulfilling and resilient life.

Tool 7, 8 & 9

Grit, Willpower & Alter Ego:

Hardening Your Mental Strength

Grit and willpower, the key ingredients to becoming Fit, Focused, Ready. Grit and willpower are like mental armor that help you weather any storm. Although often used interchangeably, they have unique and complementary roles in building your mental strength.

Grit is the ability to withstand tough and unpleasant situations over and over again. It's about sticking with your goals and not giving up, even when the going gets tough. Willpower, on the other hand, is all about making the right choices and decisions, especially when they're tough. It's saying no to that slice of cake when you're trying to eat healthily, or pushing yourself to do that extra lap even when you're already tired.

Grit and willpower are like muscles that need to be exercised regularly to become stronger. And the good news is that life offers you countless opportunities to practice them every day. You just need to be mindful of your thoughts and apply these skills when the situation arises.

To boost your grit and willpower, attach them to your self-image and alter ego, the superhero version of yourself. Visualize yourself as a machine with massive willpower, who can drive through any challenge. This will help you strengthen your mental armor and become unstoppable.

Let's break down each concept and expand on them further:

Grit

Grit can be defined as the ability to persist and maintain effort towards long-term goals, even in the face of adversity or obstacles. It's about having the mental toughness and perseverance to stick with something even when it's hard or uncomfortable. Grit is not something you're born with; it's a skill that can be developed and strengthened over time.

One way to increase your grit is to set specific goals that require sustained effort and practice. This could be anything from training for a marathon to learning a new language. When you encounter obstacles or setbacks, use them as opportunities to build your grit muscle by persevering and pushing through the discomfort. Also, keep track of your progress and celebrate small wins along the way.

Willpower

Willpower is the ability to resist short-term temptations and make choices that align with your long-term goals. It's about having the self-discipline to delay gratification and make decisions that are in your best interest. Willpower is not a finite resource; it can be strengthened with practice.

To increase your willpower, start by setting clear goals and establishing a plan to achieve them. This will help you stay focused and motivated. When you're faced with a temptation, remind yourself of your long-term goals and the reasons why you're pursuing them. Also, try to eliminate or minimize temptations in your environment to reduce the need for willpower.

Alter Ego

An alter ego is a persona that you create to embody the qualities and traits that you want to embody in a particular context or situation. It's a way to tap into your own inner strengths and resources and channel them in a more focused and intentional way. Developing an alter ego can help you overcome self-doubt and fear, and empower you to take on challenges with confidence and conviction.

To create an alter ego, start by identifying the qualities and traits that you want to embody in a particular context or situation. This could be anything from confidence to focus to resilience. Then, create a persona that embodies those qualities and give them a name, backstory, and physical characteristics. Use this alter ego to help you tap into your own inner strengths and resources and channel them in a more focused and intentional way.

Mastering these tools takes time and practice, but they are essential in your arsenal for conquering the mental game. With these at your disposal, you're not just training your body; you're fortifying your mind. So, gear up, soldier. It's time to strengthen that mental muscle.

Real World Example:

imagine facing a challenge that tests you to your limits – perhaps it's a physically grueling endurance race, a high-pressure professional deadline, or a personal goal that demands every ounce of your strength and determination.

First, you summon your Willpower. It's the initial spark, the force that gets you moving when every part of you resists the start. This Willpower is like the ignition of a powerful engine, propelling you forward with a clear intention. You remind yourself of your commitment, the reasons why you started this journey. With every step, pedal, or task completed, it's your willpower driving you, keeping you on track despite the temptation to quit or procrastinate.

As the challenge intensifies and the initial surge of willpower begins to wane, your Grit comes into play. Grit is your endurance in the face of adversity, the tenacity to keep going when things get tough. It's not just about brute strength or sheer stamina; it's the mental toughness that tells you to push through the fatigue, the discomfort, the doubt. This Grit is what keeps you moving forward when Willpower alone isn't enough. It's the voice inside that says, "I can do this, no matter how hard it gets."

But then, you reach a point where even Grit seems to falter. You find yourself in the depths of the challenge, a point so testing that it feels almost impossible to continue. This is where your Alter Ego comes into its own. You tap into this powerful inner persona, the part of you that knows no limits, that thrives on challenge, and turns adversity into fuel. This Alter Ego is fearless, unstoppable, and incredibly resilient. It's a version of yourself that transcends ordinary capabilities.

With the emergence of your Alter Ego, a remarkable transformation occurs. What once seemed insurmountable now feels achievable. You're not just enduring; you're dominating the challenge. Your Alter Ego doesn't just carry you through; it revels in the toughness of the situation, drawing strength from the very adversity that seeks to bring you down. This is where true resilience is forged, in the fires of what seems like an impossible struggle.

Together, Willpower, Grit, and the Alter Ego form a formidable trio in your mental arsenal. Willpower kicks off the journey, Grit sustains you through the hardships, and the Alter Ego powers you through the darkest hour, leading you to triumph over challenges that once seemed beyond your reach. This combination doesn't just help you survive tough situations; it transforms you, making you stronger, more resilient, and ready to face whatever comes next with newfound confidence and strength

Forging Resilience:

The Unified Force of Mental Fortitude

In conclusion, your mental strength indeed resembles the pieces of a puzzle or the layers of an onion. Each individual piece or layer, while valuable in its own right, might not seem overwhelmingly powerful or effective. However, when you combine these elements, they create a synergistic effect, revealing a complete, cohesive picture of mental resilience and strength.

Consider how each element interconnects and amplifies the others. Your mindset and mindfulness work in tandem; mindfulness grounds you in the present, helping you to become aware of your thoughts and emotions, while your mindset uses this awareness to steer these thoughts towards positive and productive pathways. This harmony between being present and purposefully directed forms the foundation of your mental strength.

Similarly, your belief is intricately linked to your self-visualization. The strength of your belief in your abilities and potential is fueled by the vividness and clarity of how you visualize yourself in the present and the future. As you see yourself overcoming challenges and achieving goals, your belief in these visualizations' reality grows stronger.

Then there's the dynamic relationship between your self-visualization and your willpower. The clearer and more compelling your visualization of who you are and who you want to become, the more fuel you have for your willpower. This willpower is what initiates action, driving you to start and persevere through challenges.

Your Grit is the enduring force that keeps you pushing through the toughest moments, complemented by the transformative power of your Alter Ego. This Alter Ego is like a secret weapon, emerging at crucial moments to provide an almost superhuman strength and resilience.

When you skillfully employ all these tools – Mindset, Mindfulness, Belief, Self-Visualization, Willpower, Grit, and your Alter Ego – you unlock a comprehensive mental strength that is far greater than the sum of its parts. It's a holistic approach where each component supports and enhances the others, equipping you with a robust mental framework to tackle any challenge, achieve your goals, and realize your fullest potential.

Ultimately, the game is to use all these tools at your disposal, not in isolation, but as a unified front. This integrated approach enables you to navigate life's complexities with a resilient and empowered mindset. With these tools harmoniously working together, you're not just surviving challenges; you're thriving through them.

Mastering Simplified Fitness

Fitness has become one of the most unnecessarily complicated topics on the planet. It should be so straightforward that anyone would know what to do to get fit. However, the fitness industry has done a fantastic job of creating a ton of needless confusion. But is it all their fault? No. Most people have no idea what they want in terms of fitness, so they jump from one routine to another, not sticking to anything long term, and thus never seeing lasting results. When, in reality, most people simply want to look decent at the beach and avoid having a lumpy, bumpy body. I learned a long time ago that being fit was pretty easy: do a few things here and there, and you're good. The less complicated, the better. Of course, once you have a specific goal and direction, pursue it full speed. But if not, don't overcomplicate things. I have been taking this approach for the last 15 years, and it works. Keep it simple, and let your mind do the rest. This book is a simplified exercise guide to eliminate the confusion of fitness and get you in the best shape of your life. So, you can focus on your goals and function at your best.

I will show you the simple workouts that I personally use to stay fit, which you can do at home with no gym equipment except for a pull-up bar and running shoes. That's it!

Your own body weight is your best friend when it comes to home workouts.

The workouts in this book are simple to understand and do. But remember, simple does not mean inherently easy. For instance, take the pushup: probably the most underrated exercise on the planet. But have you ever tried to do 100 pushups at once? Or even 50?

Simple equals success, though simple does not mean easy.

The point is to simplify the whole process of fitness. By removing complexity and confusion, there should be no confusion at all. Simplify the routine, eliminate the machines, and get after it.

"Get in the best shape of your life and never step foot in a gym."

The Push Up

Push-ups are one of the most celebrated bodyweight exercises and have been used for centuries to build strong, capable bodies. They are categorized as an upper-body pushing exercise, characterized by a horizontal pushing motion. This differs from vertical pressing movements, like an overhead press, and offers unique benefits.

Push-ups are excellent for everyone, from beginners to advanced athletes. Being a bodyweight exercise, they can be performed anywhere, making them convenient for travel or training in less-than-ideal spaces. They are one of the most versatile ways to train the upper body, adaptable to various fitness levels.

What Muscles Do Push-Ups Target?

Primarily, push-ups work the chest, shoulders, arms, and core. Specifically, they are fantastic for building the pectoralis major, triceps brachii, anterior deltoid, and rectus abdominis. Although known for enhancing the chest and arms, push-ups also require significant core engagement for stabilization during each repetition.

How to Perform a Push-Up

The setup and technique for a push-up can vary, but here's a general guideline:

1. Begin in a high plank position, forming a straight line from your head to your heels.
2. 'Grip' the floor with your hands positioned slightly wider than shoulder-width, fingers pointed forward or slightly outward.
3. As you flex your elbows, lower your body towards the floor, maintaining a rigid posture.
4. Gently touch your nose and chest to the floor. (Going this low to the floor is optional)
5. Push away from the floor, extending your elbows to return to the starting position.
6. Repeat for the desired number of repetitions.

Note: In a standard push-up, the upper body lifts approximately 65% of the total body weight with each repetition.

Common Mistakes to Avoid:

Avoid common mistakes such as flaring your elbows, dropping your head, or not fully extending your arms. Ensure your core remains engaged to prevent your hips from sagging or rising too high.

Push-ups are a fundamental exercise with variations to suit all fitness levels. Incorporating them into your routine can lead to significant improvements in strength and muscular endurance.

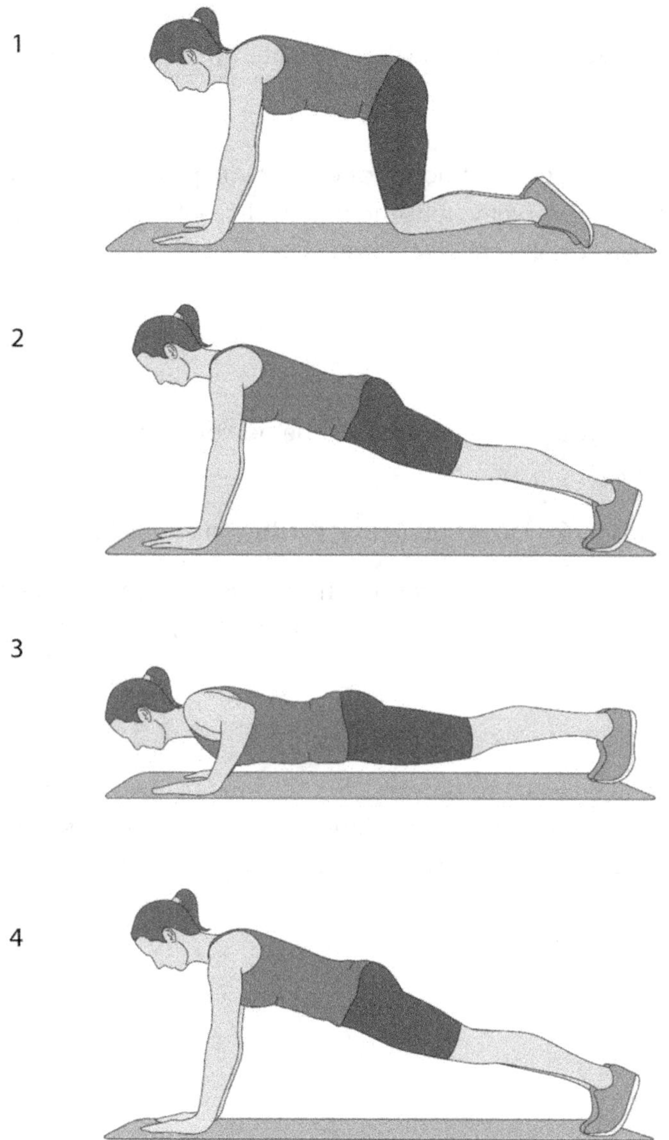

Choosing a Suitable Push-Up Variation for Beginners

For those new to push-ups or who lack the strength for a full push-up, a simple modification can pave the way to success: elevate the hands above the feet.

This adjustment decreases the amount of weight you push and reduces the exercise's demands on the core. Everyday household items like kitchen chairs, coffee tables, or a staircase are perfect for elevating your hands.

By the Numbers:

Elevating the hands by 12 inches decreases the percentage of body weight pressed to approximately 55%.

Elevating the hands by 24 inches reduces it further to about 41%.

As you build strength and become more efficient, you can gradually lower your hands towards the floor. This progression adds weight to the movement and continuously challenges your body.

Beginners should ideally aim to progress to the standard two-arm push-up, where both hands and feet are in contact with the floor. This progression ensures a gradual increase in strength and ability, leading to the successful execution of a full push-up.

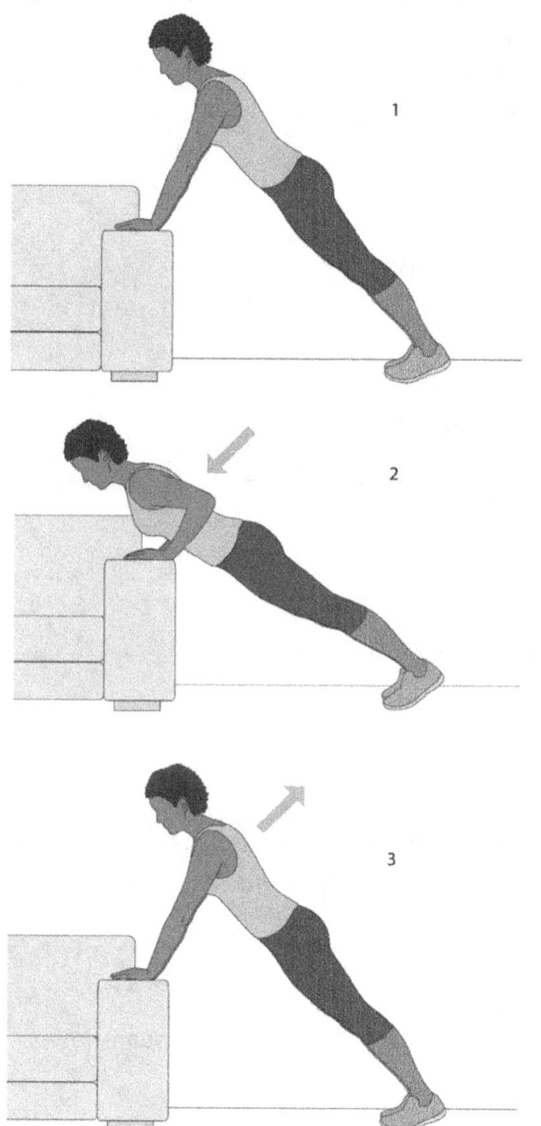

1
2
3

Intermediate / Advanced Push-Up Variations

Once you've mastered elevated push-ups, it's time to move on to standard or regular push-ups. Begin with 3 sets of 10 repetitions (30 reps in total). Note that 'reps' is short for 'repetitions'. As your strength and endurance increase, gradually add more volume to your routine. Essentially, aim to do more push-ups than you're currently doing by adding extra reps to each workout or increasing your total daily count. For example, instead of doing 3 sets of 10 reps, you can progress to 5 sets of 10 reps, bringing you to 50 reps.

Challenges to Push Your Limits:

Challenge 1: 4 sets of 25 reps.

Challenge 2: 1 set of 50 reps.

Challenge 3: 3 sets of 30 reps.

Challenge 4: 2 sets of 50 reps.

Challenge 5: 1 set of 100 reps.

Advancing the Difficulty:

Adjust the Speed: Alter the pace of your push-ups. Slow down to increase time under tension, enhancing strength and muscular endurance, or speed up to train for explosiveness.

Challenge: Spend sixty seconds completing a single push-up.

Elevate the Feet: Raising your feet above your hands shifts the weight and alters the push-up angle, increasing the challenge. Placing the feet 12 inches above the hands increases the loading by about 5%. Raising them to 24 inches increases it by approximately 10%.

Push-Ups for Performance and Fitness

Push-ups stand out as one of the most versatile and effective upper body strengthening exercises. Their importance in a fitness regimen is immense. The convenience of being able to perform push-ups anywhere means you always have the opportunity to engage in some quality pressing work. Regardless of your current workout routine, integrating push-ups can continually add significant value, enhancing overall upper body strength and fitness.

Chin-Ups

(Using a Pull-Up Bar)

The Chin-up is a functional strength exercise that uses your entire body weight, making it excellent for building core strength and increasing muscle mass.

What is a Chin-Up?

A Chin-up is a vertical pull exercise performed from a dead hang with straight arms, using an underhand grip. The motion involves pulling up vertically until the chin rises above the hands, followed by a controlled descent back to the starting position.

Note on Shoulder Issues:

The joint-friendly underhand grip of a chin-up may be the modification you need to start training vertical pulls, especially if you have shoulder concerns.

The most crucial aspect of the chin-up is the hand position. Using an overhead bar (a pull-up bar) in an underhand, supinated position (palms facing towards you) engages the biceps more significantly.

Muscles Worked in Chin-Ups:

Chin-ups target several muscle groups, most notably:

- Biceps
- Latissimus Dorsi (Lats)
- Rear Deltoids
- Abdominals
- Middle and Lower Trapezius
- Forearms (fantastic for improving grip strength endurance)

Doorway Pull-Up Bar:

A doorway pull-up bar is an ideal piece of equipment for any home or apartment gym. This versatile tool wedges securely into a doorframe and can support body weight and more.

How to Perform a Chin-Up:

1. Begin by grasping the pull-up bar with both hands, shoulder-width apart, palms facing toward you (underhand grip).
2. Keep your feet slightly off the ground, with knees either flexed or straight, achieving a dead hang position.
3. Engage your muscles to pull your body upward until your chin clears the bar, keeping elbows close to the rib cage.
4. Slowly reverse the motion, lowering yourself back to the dead hang position.

This completes one full repetition of a chin-up.

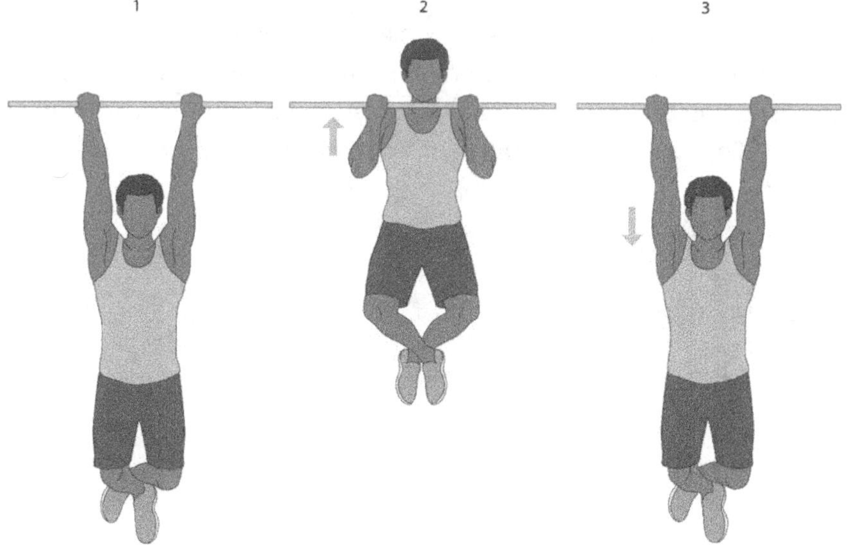

1
2
3

Chin-Up Variations for Beginners to Advanced

- Assisted Chin-Ups (decreased bodyweight demand)

- Bodyweight-Only Chin-Ups (using full body weight)

Assisted Chin-Ups:

Assisted chin-ups are designed to make the exercise more accessible by reducing the weight you need to lift in each repetition. This variation is especially beneficial for beginners or those building up to a full bodyweight chin-up.

Resistance Band Assisted Chin-Ups:

Using an inexpensive rubber resistance band is a great way to assist with chin-ups. Simply stretch the band around the pull-up bar, then bring it down and loop it around your foot. This setup uses the elasticity of the band to support some of your body weight, making it easier to pull yourself up.

The resistance band effectively reduces the weight you need to pull, allowing you to focus on form and gradually build the strength required for unassisted chin-ups. As your strength increases, you can use bands with less resistance, progressively working your way up to performing chin-ups with just your body weight.

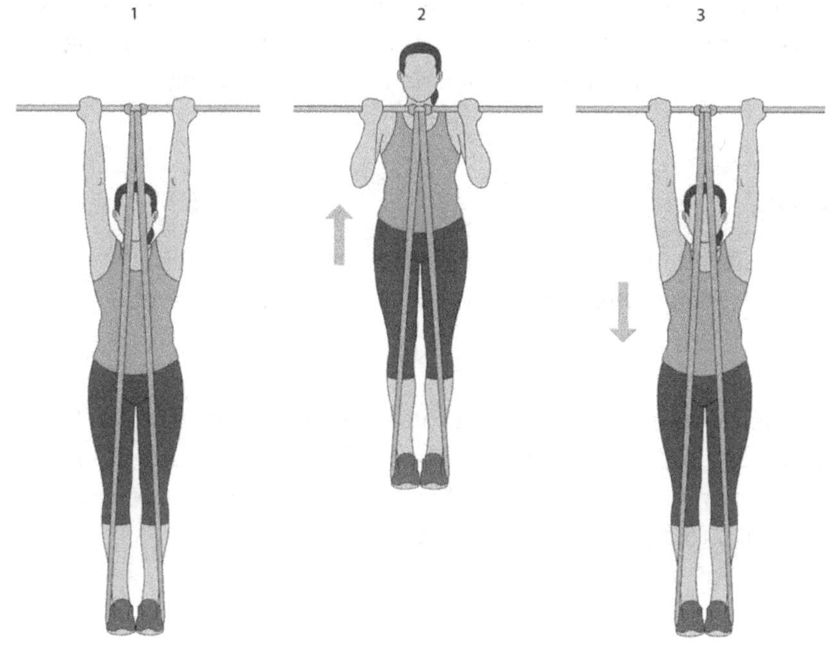

1
2
3

Bodyweight Chin-Ups:

Beginners should set a goal to progress from assisted chin-ups to full bodyweight chin-ups. Achieving a chin-up using your full body weight is a commendable feat and requires significant strength and technique.

Execution of Each Repetition:

Each repetition should be performed with a pull to the top, followed by a very brief pause. Then, ensure a controlled and steady lowering back to the starting position. This method ensures maximum muscle engagement and development.

Reps and Sets:

Once you've mastered the chin-up technique, the next question is, 'How many sets and reps should I do?' The answer depends on your current fitness level.

For most people, starting with 3 sets of 5 to 8 repetitions is ideal. If you find this too challenging at first, don't be discouraged. Remember, the primary goal is to build strength at your own pace, not to compete with others. As your strength increases, so too will your ability to perform more repetitions.

This gradual approach allows you to safely and effectively increase your strength and endurance, eventually leading to more reps and sets as part of your regular fitness routine.

Pull-Ups

(Using a Pull-Up Bar)

Like chin-ups, all you need to start building pull-up performance is access to a horizontal bar.

Many people ask about the difference between chin-ups and pull-ups. The primary distinction lies in the hand position on the bar. Pull-ups are performed with an overhand or pronated grip, while chin-ups use an underhand or supinated grip. This difference in grip alters the primary muscles engaged during each repetition, and consequently, the level of difficulty. Generally, pull-ups are considered more challenging than chin-ups.

What is a Pull-Up?

Pull-ups are a closed kinetic chain exercise. You'll begin with both hands on the pull-up bar, positioned about shoulder-width apart, palms facing away from you. The exercise involves pulling yourself up to the bar and then lowering back to the starting position. Pull-ups, like chin-ups, are performed in a vertical motion.

Pull-ups are exceptional for strengthening the back, arms, shoulder girdle, and forearm muscles. Due to the difference in hand position, pull-ups tend to be a more strenuous exercise compared to chin-ups. They require minimal equipment and can be performed anywhere there's an overhead bar.

Athletes have long relied on pull-ups to build functional upper body strength and endurance.

What Muscles Do Pull-Ups Train?

Pull-ups are one of the best functional strengthening exercises, targeting some of the largest muscles in the body, including the lats.

Primary working muscles include:

- Latissimus Dorsi: A large, flat muscle covering the middle to lower back, often referred to as the lats.
- Brachialis: An elbow flexor muscle.

Secondary muscles include:

- Trapezius: Located in the upper back.
- Rhomboids: Two muscles on either side of your upper back.
- Biceps Brachii: The large muscles on the front of your upper arms, commonly known as the biceps.

It's important to note that exercises like pull-ups and chin-ups, which involve extended durations of hanging, also help to increase grip strength, an important attribute in everyday life.

Pull-Up Technique:

Here's how to execute the traditional pull-up technique:

1. Start in a dead hang position with your palms facing away from you, hands about shoulder-width apart or slightly wider.
2. Depending on the bar's height, your knees can be flexed or straight.
3. Keep your chest up and core engaged. Pull your body as high as you can, maintaining a straight line from your shoulders to your knees.
4. Lower yourself back to the dead hang position, ensuring your body remains rigid and straight throughout the movement.

This completes one full repetition of a pull-up.

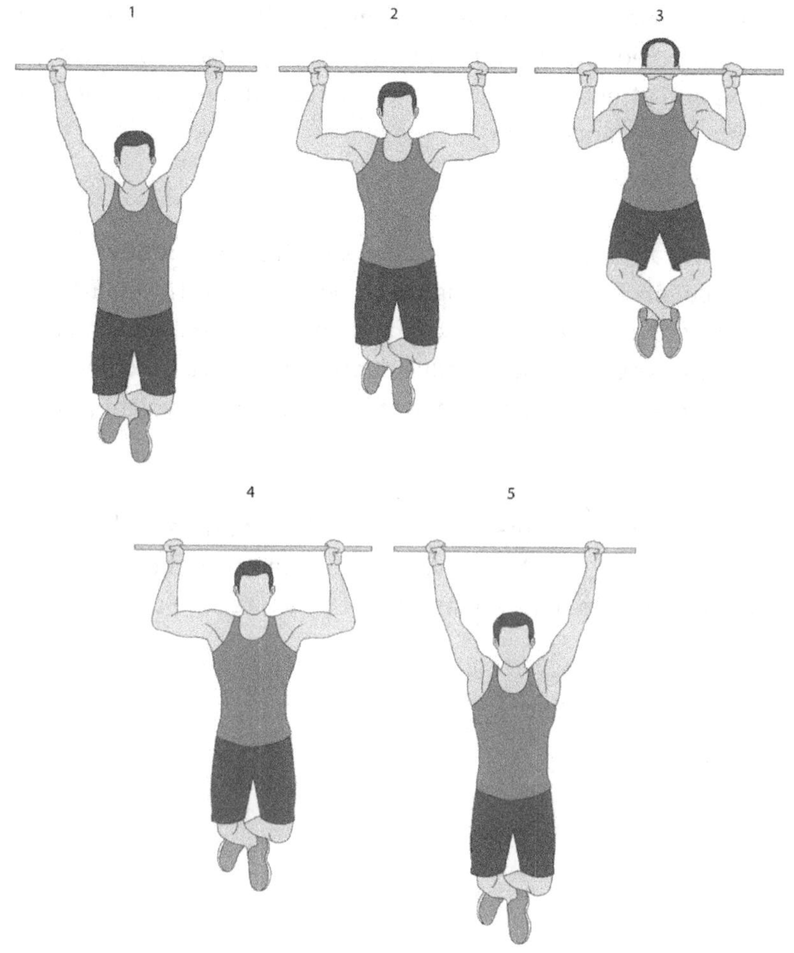

Pull-Up Variations for Beginners

For beginners, the pull-up can be an overwhelmingly difficult exercise. The pronated hand and arm position required for pull-ups create a significantly greater challenge. However, a simple and effective modification can make the exercise more accessible: introducing a rubber resistance band.

By wrapping the band around the overhead bar and stretching it down to loop around your feet, you effectively reduce the weight you need to pull. This adjustment is a fantastic way for beginners to acclimate to the demands of pull-ups and to build the necessary strength. As your body gradually adapts to the stress and becomes stronger, you'll find yourself progressing towards performing a full bodyweight pull-up.

Remember, consistency is key to making progress. Keep putting in the effort, and you'll see results. Regular practice, combined with the assistance of the resistance band, will steadily enhance your pull-up ability, leading you to master the unassisted version of the exercise.

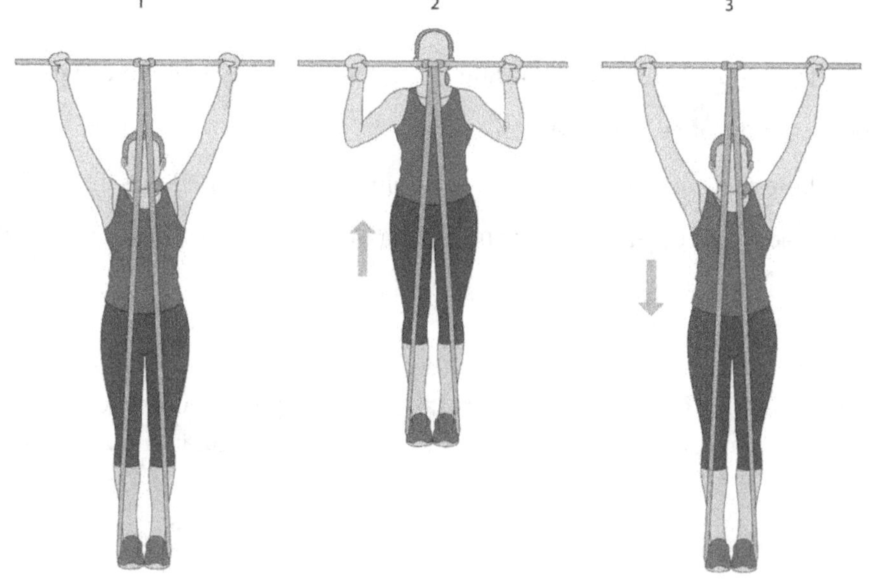

1
2
3

Intermediate / Advanced Pull-Up Training

As you progress to intermediate and advanced levels, the focus should shift to building up volume with bodyweight-only pull-ups.

Once you're able to comfortably perform three sets of 8-10 unbroken repetitions, it's time to increase the challenge. Here are a few ways to do this:

- Aim for 20–30 repetitions in a single set. This increase in volume significantly boosts endurance and strength.
- Combine pull-ups with push-ups: Try doing a set of 10 pull-ups immediately followed by 20 push-ups, without resting in between. Complete three sets of this combination to really push your limits.

By continually increasing repetitions and integrating other exercises, you'll experience firsthand why pull-ups are such effective total body changers. This approach not only enhances upper body strength but also improves overall muscular endurance and resilience.

The Plank

The plank is an excellent core stability exercise that can enhance performance and help prevent injuries. Known for increasing abdominal strength, building endurance, and improving functional fitness, the plank has direct relevance to daily life activities and sports performance.

What is a Plank?

Planks are a core-strengthening exercise that emphasizes stability. The most commonly recognized form is the prone position, with the chest facing the floor.

For beginners, it's recommended to perform the plank statically, without movement. You assume the prone position and hold it for a set duration. Maintaining alignment in this position strengthens and stabilizes the core.

Benefits of Planks:

- Builds core strength.
- Improves core endurance.
- Increases neuromuscular control.
- Trains proper muscle recruitment.
- Burns calories.
- Offers benefits that carry over to other exercises.
- A bodyweight exercise that can be performed anywhere.

Muscles Involved:

- Rectus Abdominis.

- External and Internal Obliques.
- Gluteus Maximus.
- Quadriceps.

Plank Technique:

1. Start with your body extended, toes and elbows on the floor. Your head and neck should be relaxed, and you should be looking at the floor. Position your forearms underneath your shoulders, facing forward.
2. With only your forearms and feet touching the ground, keep your body straight, rigid, and in line.
3. Hold the position for 10 seconds to 1 minute, depending on your ability.

Maintaining proper form is crucial in the plank for maximizing its benefits and minimizing the risk of injury. As your core strength improves, gradually increase the duration of the hold.

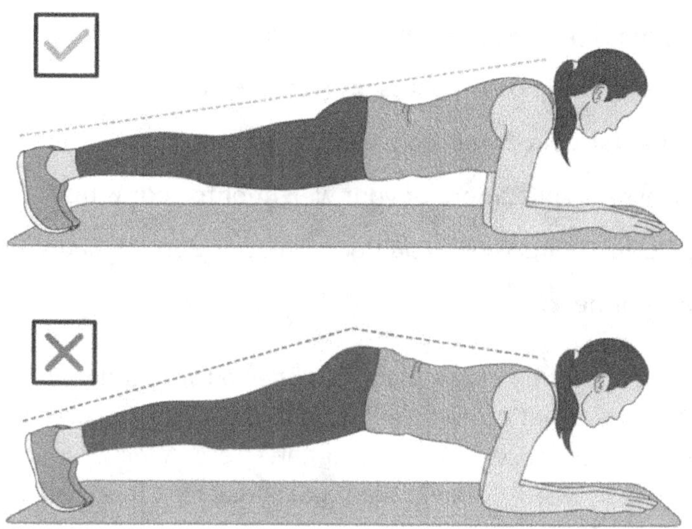

Ultimately, the hold time for a plank will depend on your fitness level, but aiming for 30 seconds is a solid initial target. Incorporate 3-5 sets per workout, ensuring an adequate rest period between each effort to allow for recovery.

Things to Avoid During a Plank:

1. **Dropping the Hips**: This is a common sign of fatigue. Keeping the hips aligned with the rest of the body ensures proper core engagement.
2. **Arching the Back**: As shown above, arching the back fails to fully engage the core and instead shifts more of your weight onto your arms.
3. **Looking Up or Tilting Your Head Back**: This position can cause unnecessary strain on your neck.

The ideal length of time for holding a plank has been a topic of debate. The key question is: at what point do the benefits start to diminish? The more you practice planks, the more your body becomes efficient at handling the stress. Aiming for a plank duration of 2–3 minutes without straining is an excellent goal. Reaching this level of endurance is a significant achievement.

The Wall Sit

The wall sit is a classic exercise primarily used for building isometric strength and endurance in the legs. While not the flashiest of exercises, it's highly effective for enhancing leg strength and endurance.

What is a Wall Sit?

The wall sit is an isometric strengthening and endurance exercise that targets the quadriceps, glutes, hamstrings, and calves. It involves maintaining a static position, effectively working out the muscles without movement. The difficulty of the exercise increases as the hips and knees approach a 90° angle. Beginners may find it challenging to hold this position due to a lack of strength and endurance.

Benefits of Wall Sits:

- Improves leg strength.
- Increases leg endurance.
- Helps build muscle.
- Conditions the mind to withstand physical fatigue.
- Protects the knees by improving quad function.
- Strengthens weak areas beneficial for squats.
- Offers many variations to suit different fitness levels.
- Can be performed anywhere.

How to Perform a Wall Sit:

1. Stand with your back against a wall, feet shoulder-width apart.
2. Press your back and head firmly against the wall. Lower your body until your hips and knees form a 90° angle, with your thighs parallel to the floor.

3. Ensure your weight is evenly distributed across your feet.

4. Hold this position for 20-60 seconds, depending on your ability.

The wall sit is a simple yet powerful exercise that can be integrated into any fitness routine to significantly improve leg strength and endurance

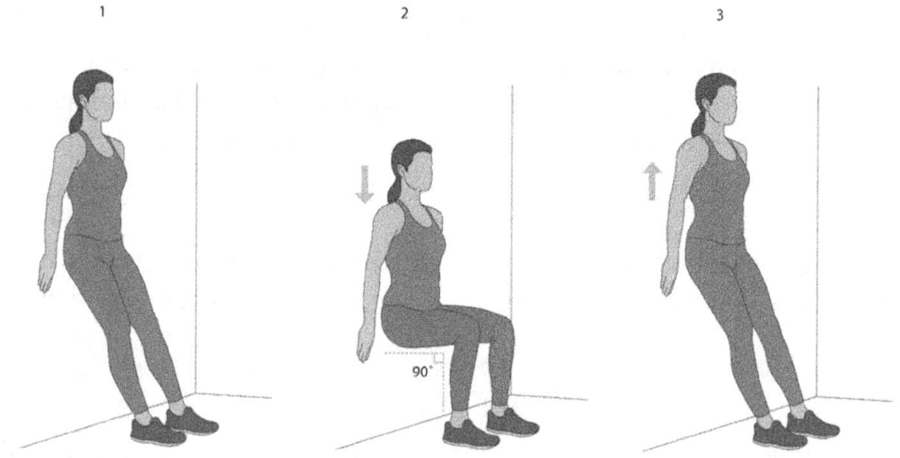

1
2
3
90°

The Wall Sit Challenge

The wall sit is not only a test of physical strength but also a challenge of mental fortitude and endurance. As you hold the position, time seems to stretch, each second feeling longer and more intense. The key is to resist the urge to move or abandon the exercise as fatigue intensifies. It's a demanding exercise that pushes you to your limits!

Typical wall sit training involves 3-5 sets of 30-60 seconds each. You can adjust the duration based on your current fitness level, either increasing or decreasing the time as needed.

To increase the challenge, try performing 3 sets of maximum time holds. In other words, maintain the position until you can no longer hold it. It's likely that the time you can sustain the wall sit will decrease with each set as leg fatigue sets in. If you're looking to build mental strength and willpower, the wall sit is an excellent choice. It's an exercise that not only strengthens your legs but also tests and enhances your mental resilience.

Running

In a world filled with expensive fitness gadgets, the simplicity of a pair of shoes, some time, and the motivation to get outside and run remains one of the most effective ways to enhance cardiovascular performance and improve overall health and longevity. Running is not only virtually free but also ranks as one of the most efficient methods for burning calories.

Runners have a 25%-40% reduced risk of premature mortality and tend to live approximately three years longer than non-runners. Any amount of running, even a modest amount each week, is better than none at all.

Let's explore some crucial running technique tips, discuss the health benefits, identify the muscles used, and describe various running levels.

The Health Benefits of Running:
- Increases cardiovascular fitness.
- Aids in weight loss and body composition improvement.
- Strengthens muscles.
- Builds strong weight-bearing bones.
- Lowers cholesterol levels.
- Improves hormone regulation.
- Boosts positive neurological functions, including cognitive function and reduced cognitive decline.
- Enhances sleep quality.
- Reduces depression and improves mental health.
- Running burns roughly 100 calories per mile, making it a cornerstone of long-term weight management and fitness.

Muscles Used While Running:

Primarily, running engages the:

- Glutes.
- Hamstrings.
- Quadriceps.
- Calves.
- Core muscles.

What's Important to Know About Running?

Developing and maintaining proper running technique is crucial for improving performance and reducing injury risk. Perfecting your running technique takes time and focus, so remain patient and dedicated to the process. Paying attention to technique makes you a more efficient runner, reduces stress on joints, and enables you to run farther and faster over time.

Running Posture:

Good running posture is essential, especially later in a run when the body is fatiguing. The ideal running posture includes:

- Maintaining a tall, upright stance.
- A slight forward lean.
- Keeping arms bent at the elbows.

Staying tall helps keep airways open, while a forward lean facilitates better hip extension and propulsion.

Arm Swing:

Arm swing significantly impacts running efficiency, providing stability and counterbalance to the leg movement.

- Keep elbows bent between 70-110 degrees.

- Hands should be loose and closer to the heart.
- Shoulders should be relaxed, with motion directed towards the body's midline.
- Find a natural arm swing that feels comfortable.

Foot Strike:

Foot strike is a significant topic in running, with varied opinions on the best approach. Sports rehabilitation therapist James Dunne from Kinetic Revolutions suggests, "There is no single perfect running technique to suit everybody. Some distance runners will benefit from a gentle heel strike, while others may be better suited to a midfoot striking running style."

Running Cadence:

Running cadence can vary from person to person. Taller individuals might take fewer strides per minute compared to shorter runners. Fitness level and power output can also influence stride rate. However, there is no optimal cadence for beginners.

Beginner Level Running:

Beginners should start slowly to avoid injury. One of the most common mistakes is running too far or too fast too soon. Gradually increasing pace and distance is key. Beginners should aim to run 2-3 days per week, with rest and recovery days in between. Over time, the body adapts, and recovery needs may decrease.

Intermediate Level Running:

Intermediate runners should build upon their established foundation, typically running 3-5 days per week. Here are a few tips:

- Take rest days seriously.
- Avoid overtraining.
- Run with a buddy or group.
- Establish a varied running regimen.

- Participate in races like 5Ks or 10Ks.

Remember, rest days are crucial. Overtraining can lead to performance issues, appetite changes, sleep disturbances, injuries, depression, irritability, and illness.

Advanced Level Running:

Advanced runners have years of experience, know their limits, and understand how to tailor their training to their goals. They often experience euphoric emotions while running, contrasting with beginners who might find each run challenging. Advanced runners can tackle any distance with appropriate training.

Running for a Lifetime:

Consistency is the key to enjoying running for a lifetime. Beginners evolve into intermediates, and intermediates become advanced runners. Enjoyment and satisfaction often increase at every stage.

So, keep lacing up those shoes and hitting the pavement or trails. Running is a journey with rewards at every step.

Cycling

Cycling is a highly popular, low-impact endurance activity that builds leg strength and enhances cardiovascular performance. With a low learning curve, cycling is accessible to all fitness levels – simply hop on the bike and start pedaling.

Benefits of Cycling:

- Increases cardiovascular fitness.
- Strengthens muscles and improves flexibility.
- Enhances joint mobility.
- Reduces stress levels.
- Improves posture and coordination.
- Lowers body fat levels.
- Alleviates anxiety and depression.
- Cycling is often a social activity, with group rides allowing cyclists of all fitness levels to enjoy the camaraderie and motivation of pedaling together.

Muscles Used While Cycling:

- Cycling primarily engages the lower body, especially the:
- Glutes (gluteus maximus).
- Hamstrings (semimembranosus and biceps femoris).
- Quadriceps (vastus lateralis, rectus femoris, vastus medialis).
- Calves (gastrocnemius and soleus).

Getting the Right Bike Fit:

A bike rarely fits perfectly right out of the box. Adjustments are typically needed for optimal comfort and performance. To avoid discomfort and maximize your cycling experience, consider getting a bike fit-test at a local cycling store. The goal is to find a bike that fits your body comfortably and promotes good riding posture.

Bike Fitting Tips:

- Select a bike frame based on your height, considering leg, torso, and arm length.
- Choose a saddle that matches your anatomy, sit-bone width, and comfort needs.
- Adjust saddle height to allow a slight bend in the knees at the bottom of each pedal stroke.
- Set the handlebar height to minimize shoulder and back tension.
- Ensure brake levers are comfortably reachable while maintaining a secure grip.
- If you experience discomfort while cycling, don't hesitate to make further adjustments to your bike setup.

Essential Safety Gear:

Before hitting the road, equip yourself with padded cycling shorts, appropriate shoes, and most importantly, a helmet. Your local cycling store can assist in selecting the right gear.

Pedaling Technique:

- Experiment with various cadences, both slow and fast.
- Focus on pulling as well as pushing the pedals.
- Keep your upper body relaxed.
- Shift to an easier gear before it becomes necessary.
- Alternate hand positions to prevent stiffness in the back and neck.

Approach to Cycling Training:

For beginners, prioritize volume over intensity. Start by cycling 2-3 times per week for 20-60 minutes at a conversational pace, aiming for a cadence of 90-100 RPM. Gradually increase your weekly riding time by about 10% every 3-6 rides. Remember, enjoyment is crucial – if you're not having fun, you might be pushing too hard.

Intermediate to Advanced Cycling:

As you progress, simply increasing saddle time isn't always enough. To continue improving, focus on increasing the workload through interval training, which involves alternating between high-intensity efforts and lower-intensity rest periods. Intervals enhance strength, endurance, willpower, and calorie burn. When you're ready to elevate your cycling, high-intensity interval training is the way to go.

Building Endurance and Strength:

Strategies for Progressing in Physical Training

To build strength, it's essential to challenge your body – this often means embracing the 'burn.' During intense physical exertion, your mind may signal that you can't push further. However, the truth is that you often can. It's about finding that extra push, whether it's one more rep or another mile. Remember, when the body reaches its limit, the mind's resilience and determination take the lead.

However, this pursuit of pushing boundaries must be approached safely. It's crucial to recognize that progress and limits go hand in hand. If you're recovering from an injury, pushing too hard can do more harm than good. Knowing when to stop for the day is a skill that develops over time.

As a beginner, my advice is to take it to the point of discomfort, but not pain. There is a significant difference between the two. Pain is direct and specific in its location – it's a clear signal from your body to halt. On the other hand, discomfort, such as a cramp, can often be worked through. Always listen to your body and learn to differentiate between these sensations.

With all this said, it's crucial to ease into any new activity. Develop your endurance and strength gradually. This approach not only fosters physical improvement but also ensures long-term health and fitness sustainability.

Integrating Fitness into Daily Life:

Tips for Making Fitness a Sustainable Part of Your Routine

In the whirlwind of everyday life, it's easy to let fitness goals slide to the backburner. However, your desire to achieve these goals should remain a steadfast priority, adaptable but never neglected. So, how do you balance the chaos of life with your fitness aspirations? This book tackles that very challenge.

The key lies in simplicity and efficiency. Fitness routines should be straightforward and brief, fitting seamlessly into your daily schedule, except for one crucial session each week: the key workout. This workout is where you give it your all, and it should be scheduled at a time when you're unhindered by other commitments. For me, Saturday mornings were sacred for this purpose. I structured my week so that nothing interfered with this pivotal workout.

But remember, not every workout needs to be lengthy or intense. The majority of your exercises can be concise, fitting into a 20-minute window. This approach respects the reality of busy schedules. As for the frequency, I found that working out three days a week plus one additional day on the weekend was sufficient to see the results I desired. Whether it's Saturday or Sunday that works best for you, the choice is yours.

The key takeaway? Never lose sight of the fact that fitness is a priority. It deserves a dedicated place in your life. By aligning your routine with this principle, you ensure that fitness becomes a natural and non-negotiable part of your daily existence.

Fitness Section Conclusion:

Ending Notes

As you begin to integrate the exercises from this guide into your daily routine, it's essential to hold onto a few key principles:

Simple Does Not Mean Easy: The simplicity of the exercises outlined in this guide is designed for accessibility and clarity, not to imply a lack of challenge. Embrace the simplicity, but prepare for the effort they require.

Progress Takes Time: Fitness is a journey, not a sprint. Each day, you are laying another brick in the foundation of your health and well-being. Be patient and consistent; transformation doesn't happen overnight.

Trust the Process: There will be days when progress seems slow or even non-existent. During these times, trust in the effectiveness of these time-tested exercises and the principles behind them. Consistency in following this guide will yield results.

Persevere for Dramatic Change: The changes you seek in your fitness and overall health are within reach. Keep plugging away at the exercises, even on days when motivation is low. Over time, you will witness a dramatic transformation in your physical abilities, appearance, and mental resilience.

Motivation and Commitment

Remember, true motivation isn't just about pushing through the workouts when you're feeling enthusiastic; it's about committing to the hard work even on days when motivation seems scarce. It's about finding that inner drive to continue, regardless of external factors or fleeting emotions.

Embrace the Challenge

Embrace the challenge laid out in this guide. Commit to the workouts, invest the time and effort, and you will see the results. This isn't just about physical fitness; it's about cultivating a mindset of discipline, resilience, and persistence that will benefit every aspect of your life

Mastering a Simplified Diet:

Only Good Options

Navigating the diet landscape is like walking through a minefield – one wrong step and boom, you're off track. I've been down every diet road imaginable, from all-fruit to all-meat and everything in between. It's a circus out there with conflicting 'expert' opinions – one minute something's a killer, the next it's a miracle cure. Amidst this chaos, trying to figure out what to eat can feel like a losing battle, especially when your own cravings are laying traps for you 24/7.

I faced this head-on while training for marathons and triathlons, where eating right wasn't just a choice, it was a necessity. That's when 'Only Good Options' came to life – a no-nonsense approach born out of necessity and simplicity. It's built on two pillars:

1. Know the Good Stuff: Understanding what's healthy is step one. It's about separating the nutritional champs from the junk.

2. Outsmart Your Cravings: Let's face it – if tasty temptations are lurking around, your brain's going to eventually win that battle. So, what's the fix? Clear out the junk food and plan for those times when you want to indulge.

That's exactly what I did, and guess what? It worked wonders. I ditched the 'normal' diet for something that made sense to me. And in this section, I'm going to lay it all out – the 'Only Good Options' strategy, plain and simple.

Step #1

The Clean Out!

The first step in Ony Good Options and in your journey toward a healthier you is "The Clean Out," a critical and transformative process that requires both determination and action. It's an intentional clearing of your food environment, requiring you to prepare with a trash bag or donation box in hand, ready to remove items that don't support your health objectives. As you meticulously inspect every item in your refrigerator and pantry, you must make the tough decision to discard anything that represents old, unhealthy habits — particularly sugary snacks, processed meats, and high-fat foods. Scrutinizing labels becomes key; any product high in sugar, saturated fats, or a myriad of additives should be eliminated without hesitation.

This purge, while seemingly ruthless, is essential. It ensures that when hunger strikes, your only available choices are those that will nourish and benefit your body. The act of reorganizing your space is just as important, making it visually appealing and logically arranged to make reaching for healthy options a natural reflex.

The benefits of The Clean Out extend far beyond the immediate satisfaction of a tidy kitchen. It's about eliminating temptation, promoting healthier eating habits, and encouraging mindfulness around food choices. It helps in reducing waste by keeping your kitchen stocked only with items you need and use, which also contributes to saving money by avoiding unnecessary purchases. With fewer unhealthy items at hand, you'll likely explore new recipes and healthier meals, enhancing your culinary creativity.

Moreover, The Clean Out often leads to a greater appreciation for local produce, as you restock with fresh options and support local farmers' markets, which tend to offer less processed and more nutritious options. This initial step is not just about decluttering; it's about instilling new, healthier habits that extend to your entire household, influencing and educating loved ones. It's a firm statement of your commitment to a new way of life, setting a tone of intent and purpose from the outset. By removing the old, you make ample room for new growth, new habits, and a new, healthier you.

Step #2

Only Good Options

Step 2 of Only Good Options is about rebuilding your pantry and fridge with healthful choices after the initial purge. This step is fundamental in ensuring that your environment is conducive to your new lifestyle. It's about making conscious choices at the grocery store and setting yourself up for long-term success. Here's what Step 2 involves:

The Shopping Mindset: As you enter the grocery store, keep the word "FRESH" in the forefront of your mind. This mantra will guide you to the perimeter of the store, where fresh produce, meats, and dairy are typically located, and away from the central aisles where processed foods reside.

Choosing Fruits and Vegetables:

Embrace a variety of colors and textures from the produce section. These foods are packed with essential vitamins, minerals, and fiber. When selecting fruit, opt for firmness, vibrant color, and a natural fragrance, indicators of ripeness and flavor. Vegetables should also be chosen for their freshness and quality — look for bright colors and crisp textures.

Selecting Seafood:

Focus on fresh or responsibly frozen seafood. Salmon and tuna are excellent choices due to their high omega-3 fatty acid content. Be mindful of the source of your seafood, opting for wild-caught or sustainably farmed options to ensure the best quality and environmental responsibility.

Picking Poultry:

Chicken and turkey are lean protein options that can be part of numerous healthy dishes. Whenever possible, choose free-range and organic poultry to avoid the antibiotics and hormones often found in conventionally farmed birds.

Dairy Decisions: (Optional)

If dairy is a part of your diet, opt for low-fat or fat-free options. However, be cautious of added sugars in products like yogurt. Dairy alternatives can also be a good option, especially for those with lactose intolerance or dairy sensitivity.

Grain Choices:

Whole grains should replace any refined grains you may have purged. Look for whole wheat, quinoa, oats, and brown rice as staples for your carbohydrate intake.

Healthy Fats:

Not all fats are created equal. Avocado, nuts, seeds, and olive oil offer healthy fats that are essential for your body's function.

Legumes and Beans:

These are excellent sources of plant-based protein and fiber. They can be used in salads, soups, and as meat substitutes in many recipes.

Herbs and Spices:

Fresh herbs and dried spices will become your best friends in the kitchen, adding flavor without the need for excess salt or fat.

Beverage Choices:

Replace sugary drinks with water, herbal teas, or infused waters. Keeping hydrated is key to maintaining good health.

Implementing "Only Good Options" is about creating a home environment where every choice is a good one. It eliminates the guesswork and temptation that come with having unhealthy foods in close proximity. By surrounding yourself with nutritious options, you make it easier to adopt and stick to a healthy eating pattern. This step is not about deprivation; it's about empowering yourself to make choices that benefit your body and your taste buds. With a well-stocked kitchen full of good options, you're setting yourself up for success in your health journey.

What to eat?

In this section, we will delve into the essentials of picking the freshest, most nutritious, and flavorful fruits and vegetables—a skill that will serve as the cornerstone of your healthy eating habits.

Armed with the knowledge of what to look for in terms of ripeness, texture, and quality, you'll be able to make informed decisions that go beyond the aesthetic appeal of shiny apples or luscious greens. You'll learn to discern the subtle signs that indicate peak nutritional value and taste, ensuring that every fruit and vegetable you bring into your home is loaded with the goodness your body deserves.

From understanding seasonal variations to recognizing the importance of a diverse color palette on your plate, this guide will equip you with practical tips and insights to enhance your shopping experience. Whether it's the crisp snap of a green bean, the sweet aroma of a ripe melon, or the firm press of an avocado, you'll gain the confidence to select the best the earth has to offer.

Let's step into the world of produce where every choice supports your journey to health and vitality. Welcome to the fresh beginnings of a healthier you.

Fruit Choices:

Apples:

- Selection: Firmness is crucial. Check for blemishes or soft spots. The skin should be vibrant and free from wrinkles.
- Nutrition: Rich in dietary fiber, vitamin C, and a variety of antioxidants. They also provide potassium.

Avocados:

- Selection: A ripe avocado yields slightly under gentle pressure. Check for over-softness or visible dents.
- Nutrition: High in potassium, folate, vitamin K, and healthy monounsaturated fats. They also contain more soluble fiber than most foods.

Bananas:

- Selection: They should be free from bruises. Bright yellow with small brown spots indicates ripeness.
- Nutrition: Rich in vitamin B6, vitamin C, potassium, and dietary fiber.

Grapes:

- Selection: Firm and attached to their stems. They should not be shriveled or leaking juice.

- Nutrition: Contain antioxidants like resveratrol. Provide vitamin C, vitamin K, and fiber.

Berries:

- Selection: They should be firm and vibrant in color. Check the container's bottom for mold or excessive moisture.
- Nutrition: High in dietary fiber, vitamin C, and antioxidants.

Oranges:

- Selection: They should feel heavy for their size (indicating they're juicy). Skin should be vibrant and free from blemishes.
- Nutrition: Excellent source of vitamin C, potassium, and dietary fiber.

Pineapple:

- Selection: Should emit a sweet fragrance at the base. The leaves should easily pluck from the top.
- Nutrition: Contains bromelain, an enzyme that breaks down protein. Rich in vitamin C and manganese.

Stone Fruits (Peaches, Plums, Cherries):

- Selection: Should be slightly soft but not mushy. Vibrant in color and free from blemishes.
- Nutrition: Good sources of dietary fiber, vitamin C, and potassium.

Watermelon:

- Selection: Look for a uniform shape with a creamy yellow spot. A deep hollow sound when tapped indicates ripeness.
- Nutrition: High in vitamins A, C, and B6. Also a good hydration source.

Vegetable Choices:

Asparagus:

- Selection: Bright green stalks with tightly closed tips. Should be firm and not limp.
- Nutrition: Rich in vitamins A, C, and K. Also provides folate and dietary fiber.

Broccoli:

- Selection: Tight, green florets and firm stalks. No yellowing.
- Nutrition: High in vitamins C, K, and A. Also contains fiber, potassium, and folate.

Brussels Sprouts:

- Selection: Firm, tightly closed, bright green.
- Nutrition: High in vitamins C and K, fiber, and antioxidants.

Carrots:

- Selection: Deep orange, firm, and free of blemishes.
- Nutrition: Rich in beta-carotene (which the body converts to vitamin A), fiber, and potassium.

Cucumbers:

- Selection: Firm, deep green, no wrinkles.
- Nutrition: Good source of vitamin K.

Celery:

- Selection: Stalks should be crisp, and leaves vibrant green.
- Nutrition: Good source of vitamin K, and also contains fiber and potassium.

Corn:

- Selection: Bright green husks tightly wrapped. Kernels should be plump and milky.
- Nutrition: Provides fiber, B vitamins, and antioxidants.

Eggplants:

- Selection: Smooth, shiny skin. Slight "give" when pressed.
- Nutrition: Contains fiber, potassium, and B vitamins.

Green Beans:

- Selection: Should snap easily when bent.
- Nutrition: Source of vitamins C and K, folate, and dietary fiber.

Kale:

- Selection: Deep green, crisp leaves.
- Nutrition: Extremely high in vitamins A, C, and K, and contains fiber and various minerals.

Leafy Greens (Lettuce, Spinach):

- Selection: Crisp, vibrant leaves without blemishes.
- Nutrition: High in vitamins A, C, and K. They also contain calcium, iron, and magnesium.

Peppers:

- Selection: Shiny skin, firm, and feels heavy.
- Nutrition: Rich in vitamins C, B6, and A. They also provide folate and fiber.

Potatoes:

- Selection: Firm, smooth skin free from sprouts or green spots.
- Nutrition: High in vitamin C, B6, and potassium. They also provide fiber.

Sea Food

As we dive into the seafood section of "Only Good Options," you'll discover the vast oceanic bounty that can enrich your diet with essential nutrients and flavors from the sea. Selecting seafood is not just about satisfying the palate; it's about harnessing the health benefits of some of the most nutrient-dense proteins available to us. This part of Step 2 will guide you through the complexities of choosing the freshest fish and shellfish, ensuring that you're making choices that are both beneficial to your health and responsible towards the environment.

Seafood is a powerhouse of omega-3 fatty acids, essential proteins, and a variety of vitamins and minerals that support heart health, brain function, and overall well-being. Whether you're a seasoned pescatarian or a newcomer to the delights of the deep, this introduction will pave the way for you to make the most of the seafood at your local market.

From the shimmering scales of fresh salmon to the deep hues of tuna steak, selecting the right type of seafood can be as intriguing as it is intimidating. You'll learn how to navigate the waters of wild-caught versus farm-raised, understand the significance of sustainability labels, and discern the freshest catch of the day.

We will also touch upon the concerns surrounding mercury content in certain fish and how to balance these concerns with the incredible health benefits that seafood offers. By the end of this section, you'll be equipped with the knowledge to confidently approach the seafood counter, make informed choices, and bring home the finest selections that the sea has to offer.

Let's cast our nets wide and explore the healthful and delicious world of seafood, an essential component of your journey to a healthier life.

********Mercury alert********

Some fish contain high levels of methylmercury (Mercury), which can harm an unborn child's developing nervous system, even before conception. So, if you're thinking about becoming pregnant, you should be aware of these risks and take steps to prevent exposure to methylmercury. As always, consult your doctor before making any changes to your diet.

Salmon

Salmon has healthy fats, it is good for your health, and it tastes amazing! Now, there are a few things you must decide when picking salmon. Wild caught or farm raised, organic or non-organic and what species of salmon?

Here is a little information to help you make your choice. There is no USDA organic standard for salmon. So, the word "organic" label means nothing really except that the salmon was raised in a farm. Now when it comes to wild or farmed, I go with wild. This is a personal choice based on red flags raised by environmental groups. With the overcrowding of pens, the fish are easily infected with lice and disease. Both of which can spread to wild salmon. Alaska has banned salmon farms. So, all salmon coming from Alaska is wild caught.

Types of salmon you will most likely see.

Sockeye:

Sockeye is an oilier fish with a deep red flesh and is high in heart-healthy omega-3s. With a strong flavor, it is a great choice for grilling.

King Salmon or Chinook:

The king is the largest of all the salmon and the most expensive. Valued for its high-fat content and smooth texture. The king is high in omega-3s and protein.

Coho:

Coho is lighter and has a milder tasting when compared to the king salmon. The Coho is considered a good dinner fish.

Atlantic Salmon:

this is the salmon you find most often in the seafood section of a grocery store. It is the farmed species of the northeast. It has a smooth fatty taste. The Atlantic is on the "do not touch" list of many environmental groups.

Tuna

Tuna is the most consumed fish in the US. People eat it for its reputation as a healthy food and for its delicious taste. Tuna is loaded with essential nutrients that help with overall health and fitness—being a good choice for weight loss, thanks to its high protein content and low calories. Be it canned or fresh, tuna is a good option.

There are several different options when it comes to choosing tuna. It can seem overwhelming, but I will try to break it down to the best I can.

There are 5 big commercially caught tunas. These consist of Albacore, Bigeye, Bluefin, Skipjack, and Yellowfin. From these, you can get canned or fresh tunas.

Canned tuna generally comes in 2 main options, white or light. White Tuna includes solid white and chunk white but refers only to the Albacore tuna. White has more of a milder flavor and a firmer consistency. Light tuna can be a mix of tuna species, most often the Skipjack, but may also include Yellowfin or Big-Eye. Light has a stronger flavor and is less expensive.

Fresh Tuna:

Albacore Tuna:

Sold mostly as canned white tuna but can be bought fresh as a loin. Albacore has a mild to medium flavor that can be great for grilling.

Skipjack Tuna:

Like the Albacore, the Skipjack is used mostly for canning but sold as light tuna. Fresh Skipjack has a stronger flavor and is great for grilling.

Yellowfin Tuna:

Yellowfin is often sold as frozen tuna steaks or fresh loins or steaks. A small amount is canned as light tuna meat and mixed with Skipjack. Fresh yellowfin tuna has a different look and taste from the tuna you buy in a can. It has a redder color with a sweet and mild flavor with a beef-like texture. Often served in sashimi, and sushi dishes.

Big eye Tuna:

The Bigeye, like Yellowfin is an extremely popular tuna among restaurants and grilling enthusiasts. It is often found in grocery stores as both fresh and frozen in either steak or loin form. Bigeye is also used in sashimi and sushi dishes.

Bluefin Tuna:

Also known as the King of Tuna is the highest valued of tuna species. You do not see them much in the supermarket. The Bluefin is used almost exclusively in sashimi or sushi dishes but can be found grilled in some restaurants. With a dark and fatty flesh, the Bluefin has a distinctive yet medium flavor.

Poultry

As we move into the poultry segment of Step 2, "Only Good Options," we turn our focus to the versatile and ubiquitous staples of many healthy diets: chicken and turkey. These lean proteins are not only a cornerstone of nutritious eating, but they also provide a canvas for a multitude of culinary creations. In this section, we will delve into the essentials of choosing high-quality poultry, both for its taste and nutritional benefits.

Chicken and turkey are lauded for their high protein content, low-fat profile, and their ability to be incorporated into nearly any meal — from hearty dinners to light, refreshing salads. However, not all poultry is created equal. The way these birds are raised can have significant impacts on their health benefits, as well as on the environment and animal welfare.

Here, you will learn to navigate the terms "free-range," "organic," and "antibiotic-free," understanding what these labels mean and why they might matter to you. We'll explore why the slightly higher cost of ethically raised poultry is often worth the investment, both in terms of health advantages and superior flavor.

This introduction will also offer guidance on how to assess the freshness of poultry at the market and tips for storing and preparing it safely at home. With the right knowledge, you can make poultry choices that align with your health goals, your ethical standards, and your palate's preferences.

Let's feather our nests with the best options available and ensure that when it comes to poultry, we are making choices that benefit our bodies, our communities, and our planet. Welcome to the informed and thoughtful selection of poultry — an essential step toward a healthier, more conscientious way of eating.

Chicken vs. Turkey: A Nutritional Tête-à-Tête

Both chicken and turkey are esteemed for their nutritional benefits. They are rich in protein, have minimal fat content, and are generally lower in calories, making them a favorite among health enthusiasts and chefs alike. However, if we were to delve into a comparison, turkey might edge out chicken slightly. Although the differences are marginal, turkey tends to have slightly less fat and marginally more protein per serving. But this shouldn't deter you from enjoying chicken; it's a close contest, and both birds offer substantial health benefits.

The Value of Free-Range and Organic Poultry

Choosing poultry isn't just about deciding between chicken or turkey. The method in which they are raised plays a pivotal role in determining the quality of the meat. Opting for free-range and organic poultry ensures you're selecting birds that have been raised without synthetic additives and have had the liberty to roam outdoors. This not only contributes to a more ethically raised bird but also results in meat that is tender, flavorful, and of higher nutritional value. The same ethos applies when selecting eggs; free-range and organic varieties are often superior in taste and nutrient profile.

The Perils of Conventional Poultry

While the price tag on conventionally raised poultry might be tempting, there are several underlying concerns. Numerous studies highlight the suboptimal conditions under which these birds are raised, often leading to compromised health and well-being for the animals. Crammed spaces, limited mobility, and the frequent use of antibiotics and growth hormones are common in conventional poultry farming. Consuming meat from such sources may not immediately present health issues, but the cumulative effects over time can be detrimental. For a more informed decision, it's always beneficial to delve into scientific research and understand the potential long-term implications of your dietary choices.

Step 3.

No Eating Out!

Embarking on Step 3, "No Eating Out During The Week," is a transformative phase in your journey towards a healthier lifestyle. This step is designed to shift your eating habits from the convenience of restaurants and fast food to the wholesome practice of preparing and enjoying home-cooked meals. The focus here is to take control of your nutritional intake by being mindful of the ingredients and cooking methods you use, ensuring that your diet is conducive to your health goals.

The decision to avoid dining out during the weekdays serves a dual purpose: it instills discipline in your eating routine and also nurtures a newfound appreciation for the food you prepare yourself. This section will provide strategies to overcome the temptation of eating out, which is often a major hurdle for many trying to maintain a healthy diet. By committing to this step, you will not only save money but also gain a deeper understanding of your food choices and their nutritional impacts.

In this introduction, we prepare to delve into practical tips for meal prepping, smart snacking, and creating a supportive environment that encourages cooking at home. This step is more than just a rule; it's a lifestyle change that empowers you to make better food choices by default, leading to improved health and wellbeing.

We'll explore how to plan your meals, the benefits of packing your lunch, and how to ensure that your kitchen is a sanctuary for health, flavor, and nourishment. By the end of this step, dining out will no longer be a reflex but a conscious choice for special occasions, and your kitchen will become the heart of your daily eating experience.

So, let's roll up our sleeves, sharpen our knives, and ready our pans as we take this pivotal step towards a healthier, more self-sufficient you. Prioritize Home-Cooked Meals

The commitment to a week without dining out is paramount. While the allure of a quick fast-food fix can be tantalizing, especially after a long workday, it's essential to steel yourself against these temptations and make your way home. While it might seem like a Herculean task, it's absolutely feasible.

Here are some strategies to ensure you stay on track:

1. Embrace the Lunchbox Ritual

Taking a leaf out of your school days, packing your lunch is a practice you ought to reintroduce. It's akin to the lunches our parents packed for us, albeit with healthier ingredients now. My recommendation? Prepare your lunch the previous evening. It eliminates morning hassles, ensuring you have a wholesome meal ready even if you're pressed for time or too sluggish. A forgotten lunch often paves the way for an impromptu fast-food detour. So, be proactive – make and pack your lunch!

2. Arm Yourself with Snacks

The afternoon slump often sends us gravitating towards the vending machine's siren call. Counter this by arming yourself with a nutritious snack. When you have a wholesome snack within arm's reach, resisting those chips becomes significantly easier. Some great snack choices include flavored or plain rice cakes, fresh fruits, air-popped popcorn seasoned with salt and pepper, crunchy veggies like carrots, or a trail mix (sans the candy).

3. Stock Your Car with Munchies

Your car can be the very arena where your willpower is tested the most. The sight of fast-food restaurants while driving can be overwhelmingly tempting. To thwart these urges, ensure you always have a healthy snack in your car. This foresight can be your saving grace in moments of weakness.

4. Relish Home-Cooked Delights

At home, the battlefield is mostly won. Having purged all junk food temptations, your food choices now lean heavily towards the nutritious side. That's the power of a well-stocked pantry with healthy options. Initially, the absence of junk food might feel jarring, but with time, your palate will adapt and even appreciate the wholesome change. For me, fresh fruits and cheddar rice cakes became my go-to for satiating sweet and salty cravings, respectively. Your choices might differ, but the principle remains – find healthier alternatives and relish them.

Step #4

Getting Active!

You might be thinking, "Haven't we already covered running, walking, and push-ups?" Absolutely, we have. But there's a solid reason we're revisiting them. If you ask me about the two most fundamental physical activities for weight loss and fitness, I'd still point you towards these:

- Push-ups
- Running/Walking

It's all about simplicity. Less is more here; fewer exercises mean making fewer decisions and encountering less confusion.

Remember our deep dive into push-ups in Section 2? If standard push-ups are a hurdle, switch to elevated push-ups. If running feels too much, start with walking. These exercises are adaptable, and that's where their power lies. They don't just shape your body; they sharpen your mental resilience.

Transforming Your Body into a Fat-Burning Furnace

You might wonder, "Doesn't my body already burn fat?" It does, but for many, this process isn't functioning at its peak. Our bodies tend to conserve fat and burn readily accessible glycogen (from carbohydrates/sugars) stored in our muscles. To shift this default and optimize fat burning, we need a strategic approach.

We can encourage our bodies to burn more fat through steady workouts, high-intensity sessions, intermittent fasting, and dietary changes. Though each method is effective on its own, combining them typically leads to the best outcomes.

Think back to Step 1, where we cleaned out the junk food and focused on nutritious foods. That was our first big step towards this dietary transformation.

Embracing Intermittent Fasting

Fasting might sound intimidating, but it's not about long periods without food. Instead, I recommend a 14-hour fasting window: no eating from 7:00-8:00 PM until 9:00-10:00 AM the next day. This schedule isn't a drastic departure for many but carries significant benefits, like better sleep, more energized mornings, and a body primed for fat burning.

After an overnight fast, your glycogen stores are low, setting the stage for fat burning. Start your day with a glass of water to assist fat metabolism. Then, dive into your chosen activity - a walk, a run, or a set of push-ups. Adjust the intensity and duration to fit your schedule. Even 20 minutes can be effective, with longer sessions providing added benefits.

By pairing intermittent fasting with morning physical activity, you're steering your body towards burning fat. Regularly practicing this routine increases your body's efficiency at utilizing fat, making the process smoother and more effective over time.

To cap it off, enjoy a nutritious meal post-exercise. This not only replenishes your body but also aligns with your overall fitness goals.

Step 5.

Weekends Are Free!

Welcome to Step 5, where weekends become your well-deserved break. This step is designed to offer you flexibility and a sense of normalcy amidst your disciplined routine. It's a time when you can relax your eating rules a bit and enjoy the foods you love in moderation. But before you set off to indulge, it's crucial to approach this freedom with a strategy that aligns with your overall health goals.

Understanding the Concept of Free Weekends:

Free weekends are not an excuse to abandon all the progress you've made. Instead, they're a psychological breather, giving you the chance to enjoy social meals, try new cuisines, or satisfy a craving that's been on your mind. It's about balance and not feeling deprived.

Making the Most of Your Free Weekends:

Plan Your Indulgences: Decide in advance what you will indulge in over the weekend. This planning prevents impulsive decisions and helps you savor the treats you genuinely crave.

Quality Over Quantity:

Choose high-quality experiences. If you're going to have pizza, let it be the best pizza available. The idea is to make those free meals count by focusing on enjoyment rather than volume.

Socialize and Savor:

Use the weekends to socialize and dine with friends or family. Eating in good company can enhance the dining experience, making the food even more satisfying.

Be Mindful:

Listen to your body's hunger and fullness cues. Just because it's a free weekend doesn't mean you should eat past the point of comfort. Enjoy your food, but do so mindfully.

Balance is Key:

If you know you're going to have a big dinner, opt for a lighter lunch. Balancing your meals can help maintain your energy levels and avoid excessive calorie intake.

*Reset for the Week:

As Sunday winds down, prepare to reset. Clear out any leftover indulgence foods to avoid temptation and get ready to return to your structured eating plan.

By integrating these principles, Step 5 allows you to enjoy life's culinary pleasures while maintaining the gains and goals of your health journey. Remember, the journey to wellness is a marathon, not a sprint, and allowing yourself the occasional indulgence can make the path more enjoyable and sustainable in the long run.

Step 6

Be Mindful

Given its critical role in our diet, it's worth revisiting the concept of mindfulness in the context of healthy eating. As with the mental strategies we've explored for exercise, mindfulness is pivotal in solidifying your commitment to a healthier lifestyle. It's about being fully present, engaged in the moment, aware of your thoughts and feelings without distraction or judgment.

Understanding Mindfulness in Eating:

In the realm of eating, mindfulness means tuning into hunger cues and distinguishing between emotional and physical hunger. It's about making deliberate food choices, recognizing the body's needs, and stopping when you're full. Just like the mental strength tools we discussed earlier, mindfulness in eating requires practice and awareness.

Listening to Your Body:

- Learn to recognize true signs of hunger versus those of boredom or stress. Commit to eating when you're physically hungry.
- Understand that hunger isn't just a physical sensation; it's a signal that needs mindful interpretation.

Understanding Your Triggers:

- Identify what drives you to eat when you're not genuinely hungry. Is it emotions, certain activities, or specific social settings?
- Just as we learned to tackle mental barriers in exercise, apply similar strategies to handle these eating triggers.

Incorporating mindfulness into your eating habits complements the physical fitness routines we've covered. It's about aligning your mental approach with your physical actions, ensuring that every choice you make is a step towards your health and fitness goals.

In Conclusion:

Embrace the Simplicity

"Only Good Options" isn't just a diet book; it's a lifestyle guide. It's about understanding our basic human nature and turning it to our advantage. By clearing out the bad and embracing the good, healthy eating becomes not just a possibility, but a natural way of life. So, toss out the junk, simplify your choices, and watch as healthy living becomes not just easy, but second nature. Welcome to a world where every option is a good one, and your path to health is clear and straightforward.

Conclusion and Wrap-Up:

Fit Focused Ready

Fit Focused Ready is more than a book; it's the embodiment of my life's system, crafted through real experiences and challenges. Every tool in these pages is a testament to a journey of transformation — designed to mold the mind into an unyielding ally, shape fitness into an effective tool, and simplify diet into a clear path for thriving. This is a system that transcends beyond the pages, adaptable and potent for anyone willing to embrace and understand its principles.

But the true power of "Fit Focused Ready" lies not in reading, but in doing. These are not just words; they are actions, steps, and habits to be ingrained in your daily life. This book is your guide to transformation — to build strength, maintain focus, and seize every day as a new opportunity to improve and excel.

As we turn the final page, the journey is just the beginning for you. Armed with these principles, you're set to forge your path to a healthier, more fulfilling life. This is your moment, your transformation, your chance to embody the essence of being fit, focused, and ready.

Embrace this journey, apply these lessons, and witness the remarkable transformation in your life. Stay strong, stay committed, and let's get after it. For in the end, it's about being "Fit Focused Ready" for whatever comes next. Let's make every moment count!

Bo Bland

Fit Focused Ready